Medical statistics made clear:
an introduction to basic concepts

40p

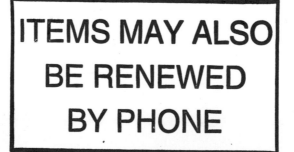

ITEMS MAY ALSO
BE RENEWED
BY PHONE

Medical statistics made clear: an introduction to basic concepts

Ashis Banerjee

Accident and Emergency Department
Whittington Hospital
Highgate Hill
London

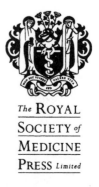

The ROYAL
SOCIETY of
MEDICINE
PRESS Limited

© 2003 Royal Society of Medicine Press Ltd
1 Wimpole Street, London W1G OAE
207 Westminster Road, Lake Forest IL 60045 USA
http://www.rsm.ac.uk

Reprinted 2004

British Library Cataloguing in Publication Data
A catalogue record for this book is available from the British Library

ISBN: 1-85315-544-6

Phototypeset by Phoenix Photosetting, Chatham, Kent

Printed in Great Britain by Bell and Bain Ltd, Glasgow

Contents

Introduction: the application of statistics to medical practice

Data collection, both for administrative and for research purposes, is ubiquitous in the health service. This data is often uncritically collected, and of varying quality, yet the inferences made on the basis of its analysis may lead to major changes in the deployment of resources or in existing clinical practice. Recognition of the validity of data collection, and understanding methods of analysis of this data are of critical importance. Appropriate data collection and analysis are especially important when assessing therapeutic advances. New or existing treatments that appear to be intuitively correct may not always turn out to be effective when one is dealing with biological variables. This has indeed been confirmed on numerous occasions when hypotheses have been tested through clinical trials.

Many, if not most, personnel working in the health service may lack a good understanding of statistical principles. In the current environment, this may prove to be a considerable handicap, especially with the advent of evidence-based medicine, and the imperative of keeping up to date with a rapidly expanding mass of literature. This book aims to provide a useful introduction to statistical principles as applicable to medical practice.

In the preparation of this text only a basic mathematical knowledge is assumed. No attempt has been made to describe the detailed mathematical analyses needed to arrive at the formulae used – indeed mathematical statistics, with its emphasis on calculus, matrix algebra and measure theory, is inaccessible to most health care professionals. The emphasis is on understanding the elements of descriptive and inferential statistics applicable to the health sciences. The principal aim is to improve the accessibility of the peer-reviewed medical literature. It is recognised that most of us will have a purely passive relationship with statistics, and that for a large majority of the important applications a grasp of the concepts is all that is necessary. Those embarking on formal research projects should, however, seek expert statistical advice at the outset.

Glossary

Algorithm: a set of instructions performed in a logical sequence to solve a problem.

Analysis of variance: a test for assessing the contribution of more than two independent categorical variables to variations in the mean of a dependent continuous variable.

Autocorrelation: a situation where a series of variables is influenced by preceding values of itself.

Average: a descriptive measure that identifies the mid-point of a set of data.

Bayes' theorem: allows revision of probabilities in the light of new information.

Berkson's bias: selection bias leading to systematic difference between hospital cases and controls in a case control study.

Bias: a systematic influence that leads to consistent over- or underestimation of the true population value, i.e. a one-sided variation from the true value. A non-random error leading to distortion of the study result.

Binary variable: two mutually exclusive variables, e.g. dead/alive, cured/not cured.

Binomial distribution: a probability distribution associated with two mutually exclusive outcomes, e.g. dead/alive.

Binomial expansion: a method of dealing with binomial variables (e.g. cured/not cured, on/off).

Bootstrap: estimation of variance and bias of an estimator by repeated random sampling with replacement from a set of observations. The bootstrap estimate is the difference between the average of a set of estimates from each sample and the original estimate.

Case-control study: an observational study in which cases and matched controls are compared with respect to exposure to the postulated causative factor.

Censoring: the loss of subjects from a follow-up study, with consequent lack of knowledge of the subsequent occurrence of the event of interest.

Central limit theorem: a statement of the fact that any distribution of sample means tends to become symmetrical and approximates to the normal distribution as the sample size increases.

Chi-square test: a hypothesis test for comparing categorical variables.

Classes: categories for grouping data.

Cluster: a group of subjects closely linked in time and/or place of occurrence.

Cluster randomisation trial: randomisation by cluster, e.g. village, practice catchment area, or school.

Cohort study: a prospective longitudinal observational study.

Collinearity: a high degree of correlation between two independent variables.

Conditional probability: the probability of an event when it is conditional on the occurrence of another event.

Confidence: the degree of certainty associated with the estimation of a variable.

Confidence interval: a range of values which is likely, with a specified degree of certainty, to contain the true population value of a variable drawn from the study sample. It is a measure of precision of the estimated value.

Confidence limits: upper and lower boundaries of the confidence interval.

Confounding variable: a variable that is related both to the exposure, usually a study factor, and the outcome, usually a disease.

Contingency table: a table that cross-classifies categorical data in rows and columns.

Co-ordinates: the values of ordinate and abscissa that define a point in a graph.

Correlation: a measure of the strength of a relationship, i.e. linear association, between two variables.

Correlation matrix: a table showing the coefficients of correlation between all pairs of variables.

Critical region: the boundary between accepting and rejecting a hypothesis.

Decision tree: a tabulation of decision alternatives and their outcomes to help identify the optimal decision, with all choices being expressed in quantitative terms.

Delphi process: an iterative qualitative forecasting process which combines individual judgements into a consensus.

Double-blind trial: a trial in which neither the subject nor the observer is aware of the allocation to treatment regimen.

Extrapolation: prediction of the value of a predictor variable outside the range of observed values of the variable.

Factorial: a declining sequence of multiplications of positive integers denoted by an exclamation mark : e.g. $n! = 1 \times 2 \times 3 \times \ldots n$.

Factorial design: an experimental design that includes all possible combinations of all levels of the independent variable, thereby allowing evaluation of all possible interactions.

Frequency distribution: (i) a plot of the values of the dependent variable against the frequency of their occurrence; (ii) the listing of all classes of grouped data and their frequencies.

Funnel plot: a plot for the detection of publication bias, in which the estimate of risk is plotted against the sample size.

Geometric mean: an average used with time series, which are growing or shrinking over time.

Goodness-of-fit test: a test to compare the expected distribution of a sample with the actual results to check conformity of the sample to expectations. It measures the degree of agreement between an empirically observed distribution and a mathematical or theoretical distribution.

Histogram: a bar chart where the area of each bar is proportional to the magnitude illustrated. It is a graphical representation of the frequency distribution of a variable.

Hypothesis test: a statistical approach to testing a theory.

Interval data: data which can be ranked by relative magnitude.

Jack-knife: a technique for the estimation of variance and bias of an estimator, based on repeated subsampling from a set of n observations, using $n - 1$ samples.

Lemma: a short theorem used in proving a longer theorem.

Linear regression analysis: a method to identify straight line relationships between two variables, where one variable is predictive of the other.

Logistic regression analysis: a method to study the relationship between two variables, where the dependent variable is a binary variable.

Logit (log-odds): the logarithm of the ratio of frequencies of two different categorical outcomes.

Markov process: a stochastic process in which the next state of an event depends on the present state only, and is unaffected by any additional knowledge of the past history of the system.

Mode: the most frequently occurring value in a set of observations.

Model: the use of numerical methods and relationships to describe real-life situations.

Monte Carlo simulation: simulation using random numbers.

Multivariate analysis: methods to analyse the effect of multiple (i.e. more than two) variables on an outcome.

Non-parametric test: a decision-making method, which does not require knowledge of the distribution of a sampling statistic.

Normal distribution: a distribution where the observations are symmetrically spread around the mean.

Null hypothesis: a statement of the absence of a true difference between two groups as the result of an intervention.

Odds: the ratio of the probability of the occurrence of an event to the probability of non-occurrence.

Odds ratio: the ratio of two odds.

One-tailed test: a statistical significance test which studies variation in one direction only.

Outlier: an extreme value in a set of observations which may distort descriptive measures such as the mean or range.

P value: the probability that the difference between two samples being greater than, or equal to, the observed difference, is due to chance alone in the absence of a real difference between the populations. Put otherwise, it is the probability that the test statistic would be as extreme or more extreme than the observed value if the null hypothesis were true.

Parameter: (i) a descriptive measure relating to a population; (ii) a summary measure of population data.

Parametric test: a decision-making method where the distribution of the sampling statistic is known.

Percentage: a proportion multiplied by 100.

Percentile: the values splitting a set of ranked observations into 100 equal parts.

Pie chart: a pictorial representation where relative magnitudes are represented by comparing areas of the slices of a pie.

Poisson distribution: a distribution modelling isolated events over time.

Posterior probability: a revised probability calculated by combining prior probability with observed results.

Power: (i) A number multiplied by itself a given number of times. (ii) The effectiveness of a statistical test, as measured by the probability of not making a type II error, i.e. the probability of rejecting a false null hypothesis.

Prior probability: an initial assessment of probability.

Probability: the likelihood of occurrence of an event expressed as the proportion of the number of occurrences of the event to the total number of possible outcomes, with 0 = no occurrence and 1 = universal occurrence.

Probability density: the frequency distribution of a continuous random variable.

Probability distribution: the listing of all possible values and corresponding probabilities of a discrete random variable.

Proportion: one number relative, or divided by, another.

Random sampling: the selection of subjects, with an equal probability of being chosen, from a large sampling frame, using a method for randomisation.

Range: the distance between the lowest and highest values in a set of data.

Regression analysis: a method to identify relationships between two or more variables.

Rejection region: the set of values for the test statistic that leads to the rejection of the null hypothesis.

Residual: the amount unexplained by any analysis.

Risk: the probability that an event will occur.

Risk ratio: the ratio of two risks, usually exposed/not exposed.

Root: the nth root of a number is represented by the factors of a number which when multiplied together n times produce that number.

Runs test for randomness: a run is a sequence of similar events.

Sample: a subset of a population.

Sample space: a collection of all possible outcomes for an experiment.

Sampling error: error resulting from the use of a sample to estimate a population characteristic.

Sensitivity analysis: an analysis where a model is re-run after alteration of a particular figure.

Significance level of a hypothesis test: the probability of type I error.

Significance test: an indicator of whether a descriptive measure (such as an average or proportion) calculated from sample data is representative of that for a population as a whole.

Skewness: a measure of the degree of asymmetry of a frequency distribution.

Standard error: the standard deviation of an estimate based on sample data. The standard error of means is the standard deviation of the sampling distribution of the sample mean.

Statistic: a summary measure of sample data.

Stochastic: a process involving probabilities.

t **test:** a test to analyse the means of small samples.

Test statistic: a statistic used as the basis for deciding whether the null hypothesis should be rejected.

Transformation: alteration of a set of numbers to facilitate interpretation and analysis.

Trend: the long-run path of a time series.

Two-tail test: a statistical significance test that studies variation in either direction from a point estimate.

type I error: rejection of the null hypothesis when it is true.

type II error: failure to reject the null hypothesis when it is false.

Z **score:** a standardised standard deviation, used to locate a point in the normal distribution. The score is expressed as the deviation from the mean in standard deviation units.

Chapter 1

Data: classification, collection, presentation

The term **statistics** refers to the collection, organisation, summarisation, presentation, analysis and interpretation of data (coded observations). An alternative useful definition is the study of populations and their variation.

Some basic relevant definitions need to be understood at the onset:

- **Population** (or **universe**) is the total collection of data, events, objects or people about whom information is required. A population may be finite or infinite, real or hypothetical. The target or reference population is the population about which it is desired to make inferences. The sampled population is the population from which a sample is taken.
- **Census** is a sample consisting of the entire population. When dealing with a large population it is expensive and time consuming to obtain census data, along with the risks of missed data and reduced accuracy owing to the logistics of the process. Furthermore, when performing quality control studies it is not permissible to use the entire population for the study. Statistical techniques are thus often concerned with making inferences on the basis of samples to reduce cost and errors.
- **Sample** is a representative subset of the population. The sampling frame is the list of units from which the sample is chosen.
- **Unit** or **element** is any individual member of the population.
- **Parameter** is a summarising value, which describes a population, i.e. a numerical characteristic of the population. It is a fixed value, which does not change from measurement to measurement.
- **Statistic** is a summarising value that describes a sample from the population, i.e. a numerical characteristic of the sample (observed data).
- **Variable** is a characteristic of the smallest sampling unit: a quantity that is measured for those units in the sample. It can take any one of a set of specified values.

Data are univariate when only one variable is measured on each unit, bivariate when two variables are measured on each unit, and multivariate when more than two variables are measured on each unit. Measuring weight alone would be an example of univariate data, height and weight together would be an example of bivariate data, and height, waist circumference and weight on each sampling unit an example of multivariate data collection.

The inherent variability in biological populations is a major reason for the need for appropriate statistical techniques in analysis of data from these populations. This implies that the characteristics of the population cannot be inferred from the characteristics of a single member of that population. The larger the population size the larger the sample size needed to determine its characteristics.

The causes of variability can be listed as:

- Random natural variability, due to physiological fluctuations and to genetic variation.
- Errors in measurement, which may be systematic (bias), random, or combinations of the two.
- Sampling error.

Classification of statistical techniques

1. **Data collection**, which is either passive (by observation) or active (by experiment). Raw data are data recorded in the sequence with which they are collected, prior to processing, i.e. grouping or ranking.
2. **Descriptive statistics**, which are concerned with the description and presentation of data. These include:
    (i)   Methods for organising sample data (e.g. tables, histograms, bar charts, pie charts, frequency polygons).
    (ii) Measures of central tendency (or location)(e.g. arithmetic mean, median, mode, geometric mean, harmonic mean, weighted arithmetic mean).
    (iii) Measures of spread (or dispersion)(e.g. range, interquartile range, standard deviation, variance, sum of squared deviation scores).
3. **Inferential statistics**, which are concerned with the drawing of conclusions about a target population based on the analysis of data obtained from a random sample drawn from that population. These conclusions may take the form of inferences or predictions about the population. Inferential statistics comprise the following elements:
    (i)   The population to be studied.
    (ii) The investigation of one or more variables of this population.
    (iii) A sample from this population.
    (iv) Inference about the population based on analysis of the sample.
    (v)   A measure of reliability for the inference.
They may be used to:
    (vi) Test the level of confidence with which a sample may be regarded to be representative of the population.

(vii) Test the probability that two separate independent samples come from the same population.

Measurements of central tendency

Arithmetic mean (average) (interval data only)

The sum of all values making up the set of observations divided by the total number of observations in the set. The Greek letter sigma, Σ, is commonly used as a summation sign, with the subscript (expression below) indicating the first item included in the summation and the superscript (expression above) indicating the last item.

It can be influenced by extreme values (outliers) in small samples of data. It is a simple calculation, but can give fractional values even with discrete data. It is the measure of central location about which the sum of squares is a minimum.

A **weighted arithmetic mean** is obtained by multiplying each individual value by a constant based on its frequency of occurrence before adding up the products, and then dividing by the sum of frequencies. The idea is to assign a weight to each value to reflect its relative importance.

Trimmed means

If stray or erroneous observations (unusually small and/or unusually large data values) are suspected one may use either of the methods described below after arranging the data in order of magnitude.

P% *truncated mean*

- Reject the highest and lowest $(P/2)$% of the observations and take the arithmetic mean of the remainder.

P% *Winsorised mean*

- Reject the $(P/2)$% highest observations and count them as if they had occurred at the highest observation still included. The $(P/2)$% highest observations are not dropped altogether but are each reduced to the highest value not trimmed.
- Reject the $(P/2)$% lowest observations and count them as if they had occurred at the lowest observation still included. The $(P/2)$% lowest observations are not dropped altogether but each increased to the lowest value not trimmed.
- Obtain the arithmetic mean of the result.

Trimmed means techniques reduce sensitivity to outliers in the data, and provide a better indicator of the central location of the data. They are reasonably efficient as an estimator for normally distributed, i.e. not skewed, samples.

Median (interval or ordinal data)

The central value, or 50th percentile, of a set of observations ranked in order of magnitude, given an odd number of observations. The median divides a frequency distribution into two halves.

If there is an even number of observations, the median is taken as the mean of the central pair. It is the same as the geometric mean with a lognormal distribution.

It is not capable of much useful arithmetic manipulation. Its value is not affected by an outlying observation, and thus is a better measure of central tendency with skewed data.

It is used in many non-parametric statistical tests in place of the arithmetic mean. It is a better measure for large data sets.

Mode (interval, ordinal or nominal data)

The most frequently occurring value of a set of observations, representing the peak of the curve describing a frequency distribution. It disregards most of the observations.

Some distributions may not have a mode, while others may have more than one. The presence of two or more modes usually indicates that the data are not homogeneous and that two or more distributions have been combined. The mode may occasionally be an extreme value where it does exist.

The mode is not capable of arithmetic manipulation. It is useful for large data sets.

Geometric mean (ratio scale data)

The nth root of the product of n values.

It can be calculated by calculating the arithmetic mean of the logarithms of the observations and taking the antilogarithm of the result. This is in effect a back-transformed mean of a logarithmically transformed variable.

The geometric mean is always smaller than the arithmetic mean. It is approximately equal to the median if the data are skewed to the right. It is not unduly influenced by extreme values, thereby reducing the effects of outliers. If any of the measurements are zero or negative it cannot be used. It is useful for situations of constant growth or constant decay, e.g. population growth studies, bacterial reproduction.

Harmonic mean (ratio scale data)

The reciprocal of the arithmetic mean of the reciprocals of individual observations. It is always smaller than the geometric mean.

Trimean

A weighted average of the median and quartiles, with the median receiving twice the weight of each of the quartiles.

An **ideal measure of average** should:

- Be easy to calculate.
- Be capable of objective definition.
- Make use of all the data.
- Be usable mathematically in other statistical calculations.

Percentiles

A percentile is a measure of location of data that provides information about the spread of data over the interval from the smallest to the largest value, i.e. the shape of a distribution.

The pth percentile divides the data set into two parts: $p\%$ of items have values less than the pth percentile, and $(100-p)\%$ of items have values greater than the pth percentile.

To calculate the pth percentile:

- Arrange the data in ascending order.
- Calculate the index i: $(p/100)n$ where p is the percentile of interest and n is the number of items.
- If i is not an integer, the next integer value greater than i denotes the position of the pth percentile.
- If i is an integer, the pth percentile is the average of the data values in positions i and $i + 1$.

Measures of spread (or dispersion)

Measures of the range

- The **range** is the difference between the largest and the smallest values in a series or distribution. It is concerned only with extreme values, and thus may be unrepresentative of the spread of items.
- The **interquartile range** contains the central 50% of a distribution. It lies between the upper and lower quartiles. It is resistant to outliers as it ignores the upper and lower 25% of the data. The 1st, 2nd and 3rd quartiles are the summary measures that divide ranked data into four equal parts. The 2nd quartile is the same as the median. It is the preferred measure of range to use with skewed distributions.
- The **quartile deviation** or **semi-interquartile range** is half the interquartile range. It is the mean of the first and third quartile values. It is the appropriate measure of range to use when the median is used as the measure of central tendency.

Measures of average deviation

- The **variance** is the average of the square of all the deviations from the arithmetic mean. This is thus expressed in squared units of measurement.
- The **standard deviation** is the square root of the variance, and is expressed in the same units as the mean. It is a measure of the spread of data about their mean, weighting each individual item by its distance from the centre of the distribution. It is a measure of absolute dispersion or variability, and is affected by the units of measurement used. The standard deviation is used in place of the variance when a measure of concentration in the same units as the random variable is desired. A small standard deviation indicates clustering of the values around the mean, while a large standard deviation indicates increased scatter of the values around the mean. Summations cannot be performed on the standard deviation, but can be performed on the variance.
- The **coefficient of variation** is the standard deviation divided by the mean, expressed as a percentage. It is a measure of relative variability, and has no units at all. It can only be calculated for ratio scale data, but helps place the standard deviation in perspective by relating it to the size of the mean. The use of the coefficient of variation allows the comparison of two standard deviations, which are in different units.

Calculation of standard deviation (root mean square deviation from the mean)

- Calculate the arithmetic mean for the sample.
- Subtract the sample mean from each value of the variable to obtain the deviations from the mean.
- Square each value of the deviation. This avoids the cancelling effects of negative and positive values.
- Add together the various squared values.
- Divide the sum of squares by $(n - 1)$, which represents the degrees of freedom, i.e. the remaining value can be calculated from $(n - 1)$ of values and the sample mean. This is the variance. The divisor $(n - 1)$ ensures that the sample variance obtained in this step is an unbiased estimator of the population variance.
- The square root of this value is the standard deviation.
- Division of the sum of squares by n is appropriate when data is available on the entire population.

The normal distribution has a range of approximately 6 standard deviations.

Coefficient of variation

This is equal to standard deviation/mean (as a percentage) It is a measure of relative dispersion in populations that have different means, and is independent of the units of measurement.
It is of some use in comparing two or more data sets.

Sheppard's correction

If the class interval size is C, then $C^2/12$ should be subtracted from the average of squares of errors before taking the square root in order to obtain the corrected standard deviation.

Standard error of the means

This is equal to standard deviation/square root of n where n is the sample size, which represents the standard deviation of a sampling distribution.

It is a measure of the precision with which the sample mean approximates the population mean.

The standard error describes the error in measurement in a hypothetical population of sample means rather than an actual sample. The size of the standard error is dependent on the variability of the sample from the parent population, and on the number of observations in the sample. If the sample size were in fact the same as that of the population, the standard error would be zero, as repeated samples would have an identical mean.

Outlier

An outlier in a set of data is an observation (or subset of observation) which appears to be inconsistent with the remainder of that set of data. It may represent a genuinely extreme value, or be caused by errors in measurement, data recording or data entry (including miscoding). Some observations may not be genuine members of the population, and are termed contaminants.

Options for the management of outliers

Outliers can either be accommodated in the statistical analysis or rejected.

- Ensure that data collection is accurate, with correction of any errors in the data by deletion or down-weighting.
- Exclude outliers to 'smooth' out the data distribution.
- Report results with data on outliers both included and excluded.
- Transform the data to 'smooth' the distribution (e.g. log transformation).
- Collect more data in order to dilute the effects of the outliers.
- Consider a different model.

Data

Types of data

Data is described in terms of variables, which define a characteristic or property which helps differentiate individual members of a sample.

Data can be classified as either qualitative or quantitative.

Qualitative variables

Nominal or categorical (classified) data

The data are categorised according to names that indicate an attribute or classification, and are represented by counts or numbers of observations in each category. These data cannot be measured or ordered. The distances between the categories cannot be defined. Indirect measures include the use of percentages, proportions, rates and ratios.

The categories are mutually exclusive, with no overlap and no intermediary values. The data cannot be subjected to arithmetical computation (e.g. addition, subtraction, multiplication, division). Examples include: sex, marital status, ethnic group, employment status, blood type.

Binary or dichotomous data

The data are categorised in one or other of two mutually exclusive categories, and are either nominal or categorical. Examples include: dead/alive, cured/not cured.

Ordinal (ranked) data

The data are organised in mutually exclusive categories. These display a logical order based on subjective ranking, using a relative scale of magnitude. The differences between adjacent categories is not equal, and the intervals are not known. The data cannot be subjected to arithmetic computation (e.g. addition, subtraction, multiplication, division).

Examples include:

- Rating or measuring scales, such as the Glasgow Coma Scale, Injury Severity Scoring Scale, Waterlow Scale, Apgar Scale, Jarman Index.
- Visual analogue scales, e.g. for pain rating.

- Staging systems for disease.
- Social class.

Quantitative variables (numerical data)

Discrete numerical data

The data can take only certain fixed numerical values, usually whole numbers (integers). These values increase in a stepwise fashion with no possible intermediate values. Ordering and magnitude are both important.

Examples include: number of children, number of patients.

Continuous numerical data

The data can take any number value within a given range, i.e. within two fixed points. There are an unlimited number of values, which may have fractional or decimal components, depending on the accuracy of the measurement system available.

Examples include: temperature, weight, height, blood pressure.

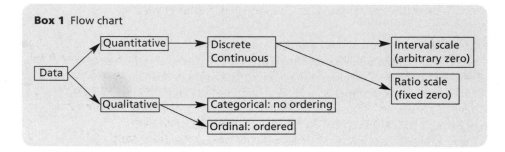

Box 1 Flow chart

Qualitative variables can be assigned numbers by the following processes:

- Coding.
- Rank ordering.
- Rating scales.
- Weighting.

Scales of measurement for variables

Any scale of measurement must be defined in terms of two fundamental quantities: the zero and the unit. Equivalence of intervals between variables is required to allow arithmetic manipulation (addition, subtraction, multiplication and division) of the measurements of a scale.

The scales listed below are arranged in ascending order of informativeness:

Nominal or categorical scale

The variables simply define categories, which describe some quality possessed by the variable, thereby allowing classification of an object, person or characteristic.

The categories may be given a non-numeric label (e.g. race, sex) or a numeric code (e.g. identification numbers for patients). There is no rank ordering of observations, i.e. no natural order. There is no absolute zero point.

Ordinal or ranking scale

The variables can be arranged in numerical order from highest to lowest value with regard to the relative amount of some characteristic that each possesses (e.g. size, value, complexity) without precise quantification of the difference between categories. Thus only the relative magnitudes of the data are known. There is no absolute zero point.

Interval scale

The intervals between observations can be expressed in terms of a fixed unit of measurement. Equal intervals are equivalent but the measurements using one set of units are not constant multiples of measurements using a different unit. The zero point is arbitrary, i.e. there is no absolute zero point. An absolute zero point refers to true and total absence of the variable under study.

Examples include certain temperature scales (fahrenheit, centigrade). Some interval scales are circular scales, such as times of day or of year.

Ratio scale

The ratio of two observations is meaningful. The zero point is well defined and fixed, i.e. there is a true zero point of origin. The zero point represents absence of the characteristic being measured. For example, in the Kelvin temperature scale the absolute zero is at $-273°C$, and represents the lowest possible temperature that could exist anywhere at all. There are equal units of measurement.

Examples include weight, distance, time, Kelvin temperature scale.

Most statistical data analysis procedures do not distinguish between the interval and ratio properties of the measurement scales.

Derived variables

These are variables calculated from the relationship between two or more independent variables:

- Ratio: expressed as a fraction or as a quotient.
- Percentage: expressed as a fraction of 100.
- Index: an average or a summation of several measurements.
- Rate.

Box 2 Choice of summary statistics

Scale	Summary statistics
Nominal	Central tendency: Mode
	There are no measures of spread
Ordinal	Central tendency: Mode, median
	Spread: Range, interquartile range
Interval/ratio	Central tendency: Mode, median (skewed data), mean (symmetrical data), geometric mean (logarithmic scale data)
	Spread: Range, interquartile range, standard deviation

Presentation of data

The organisation of raw data can be achieved according to the type of data under consideration as described below.

Discrete data
- Table.
- Bar chart.
- Pictogram.
- Pie chart.
- Graph.
- Dot plot.

Continuous data
- Grouped frequency distribution.
- Histogram.
- Stem and leaf diagram.
- Box and whisker plot.
- Lorenz curve.
- Frequency polygon.
- Ogive or cumulative frequency curve.
- Picket fence plot.

Paired data
- Scatterplot.

Exploratory data analysis

Exploratory data analysis refers to the use of graphical methods to compress and summarise data, thereby identifying properties of the data set that suggest appropriate statistical analyses and simultaneously exposing unusual features of the data set. Data exploration is essential before undertaking inferential statistical analysis.

Graphical methods of display of data are useful in the following ways:

- Recognition of the structure of, and patterns in, the data, including clusters and outliers.

- Detection of errors in the data.
- Exploration of relationships among variables.
- Assessment of the adequacy of fitted models.
- Discovery of new phenomena.
- Identification of the need for, and method of obtaining, corrective action: data transformation, collection of more data or redesign of the experiment.

The four components of exploratory data analysis include:

- Visual display of the data to suggest the appropriate statistical analysis.
- Examination of the residuals, i.e. the differences between the observed data and the fitted model.
- Re-expression of the data to simplify and improve analysis, e.g. transformations.
- Reduction of the sensitivity of the analysis and summary of the data to ensure resistance to outliers.

Table

Tables can be used both for presenting data and for interpreting data. The optimal requirements are:

- A concise, explanatory title.
- A clear indication of units of measurements.
- Clearly stated data in headed columns, with clearly labelled rows. It is easier to follow a sequence of numbers down a column, rather than across a row.
- Omitting grid lines.
- No double counting.
- Column and row totals and subtotals if helpful.
- Clear indications of the sources of data.
- Extra information as footnotes.

Bar chart

The features are:

- A discrete horizontal scale.
- A series of non-adjacent vertical bars of equal width. The bars represent the categories of a nominal or ordinal variable.
- A vertical scale starting at zero.
- The height of the bar represents the frequency of the variable.
- The bars are separated from each other to emphasise lack of continuity.
- In a component bar chart each bar is broken down into its component parts.

Pictogram

The features are:

- The shape represents the variable in pictorial form.
- With size-proportional pictograms, the size of the selected shape is directly proportional to the amount of the variable represented.
- With size-constant pictograms, a shape of given size represents a fixed number of units of the variable.

Pie chart

The features are:

- A circle is divided into sectors whose areas are proportional to the frequencies or percentages of the categories they represent. The number of sectors or slices should be between 3 and 10. The total amount of data is equal to 360 degrees of the circle.
- No scales are required.

It is difficult to compare more than one set of values and to draw very small sectors.

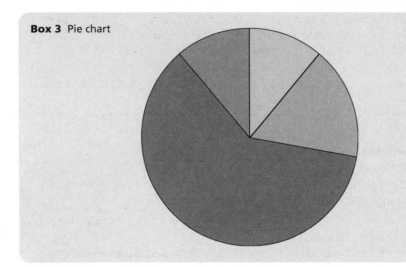

Box 3 Pie chart

Graphs

The optimal requirements are:

- A clear comprehensive title.
- The values of the independent variable are plotted on the horizontal or x axis as the abscissae.
- A vertical scale, the y axis, starts at zero and the variables on this axis are the ordinates. This variable depends on x.
- A point on the graph is defined by its abscissa and ordinate, its Cartesian or x, y co-ordinates. A line joining a sequence of points is referred to as a curve, even if it is straight. Plots may be joined by ragged, stepped or smooth lines.
- The axes must be labelled.
- The axes must not be compressed or incomplete.
- An indication of the source of the figures used must be provided.

Graph manipulation may lead to misleading interpretations, e.g. by:

- Changing the scale on one or both axes.
- Truncation of the frequency axis (i.e. starting the axis at a number greater than zero).
- Inversion of the vertical or y scale.

Logarithmic scale graphs show proportionate changes directly. Equal slopes denote equal rates of change, regardless of changes in the absolute magnitude of the variables involved. A logarithmic scale converts an exponential curve into a straight line. In logarithmic-linear (semi-log scale line graphs) graphs the x axis represents a linear arithmetic scale and the y axis a logarithmic scale.

Dot plot

This is a plot of individual values of a data set. It is useful for a small data set, with preferably under 20 observations.

- One or more categories of a non-continuous variable are plotted on the x axis.
- The range of values of the observations is plotted on the y axis.
- The numerical value of each observation, i.e. each individual data point, is located by a dot.
- Identical values of observations are plotted adjacent to each other on the same horizontal line.
- The plot can be used to show the location of data and their variability.

Grouped frequency distribution

Construction involves:

- Location of the largest and smallest observation.
- Calculation of the range.
- Use of the range as a guide to determine the number of class intervals.
- Construction of the class intervals.
- Tally of the number of observations in each class interval and conversion of the tallies to counts (frequencies).
- The modal class is the class with the highest frequency.
- Organisation of the table and provision of a title.
- Listing of the class intervals in the left column and corresponding frequencies in the right column.

Histogram

This is a pictorial representation of a frequency distribution of a random variable within a sample, in the form of adjoining rectangles.
The features are:

- The horizontal axis is a continuous scale including all the units of the grouped class intervals.
- For each class in the distribution a vertical rectangle or block is drawn from the lower class limit to the upper class limit. The base of the rectangle is the class interval. The width of the base is proportional to the width of the class interval. The vertical scale should start at zero.
- The area of the block is proportional to the frequency of the class, i.e. the number of subjects.
- The Sturges formula may help in the choice of the number of class intervals needed. The usual range of class intervals is between 5 and 15.

- It is preferable that the class intervals are equal, as then the height of each is proportional to the frequency.
- There are never gaps between the blocks because the class limits are true limits in the case of continuous data.

Box 4 Sturges formula

$k = 1 + 3.322 \, (\log_{10} n)$
where k = number of class intervals
n = number of values in the data set being studied

- A histogram with one peak is unimodal, with two peaks is bimodal, and with more than two peaks multimodal.

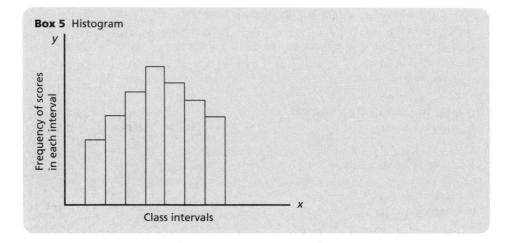

Box 5 Histogram

Frequency of scores in each interval

Class intervals

Stem and leaf diagram (J.W. Tukey)

The features are:

- Each row is a stem. The stem is the core value of the unit, i.e. the leading digit(s), or the portion of the measurement to the left of the decimal point where applicable. Generally the stem involves a power of ten.
- The stem is demarcated by a vertical ruled line, thereby leading to the listing of the stem values in a vertical column.
- The ordered sequence of digits to the right of the ruled line are leaves on the stems. These are the trailing digits, or the less significant components.
- The stem and leaf units should always be recorded.
- It retains all information on individual values, displaying all the actual data values.
- It can be used to rank order data and reveals the range of the data set.
- It provides information about the presence or absence of symmetry.
- It indicates the degree to which the data are homogeneous.

> **Box 6** Example of a stem and leaf diagram
>
> If a group of subjects with a given disease have the following ages: 42, 44, 45, 45, 51, 53, 56, 59, 60, 61, 62, 63, their ages can be represented as:
>
> 4 2,4,5,5
> 5 1,3,6,9
> 6 0,1,2,3

Box and whisker plot (J.W. Tukey)

The features are:

- Construction requires ordering of the data.
- On a linear scale vertical marks correspond to the minimum, 1st quartile, median, 3rd quartile and minimum.
- The minimum and maximum values (range) are indicated by the extremities (whiskers).
- The median (50th percentile) is indicated by a central vertical line, within the box.
- The lower and upper quartiles (25th and 75th percentiles) are indicated by the corresponding vertical ends or hinges of the box, which contains the central 50% of values. The box thereby encloses the interquartile range, sometimes referred to as the H spread. An outlier is beyond the whisker but less than three interquartile ranges from the box edge. An extreme outlier is more than three interquartile ranges from the box edge.

The box plot thus shows the centre, spread and skewness of a data set.

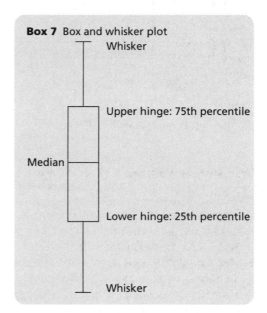

Box 7 Box and whisker plot

Whisker

Upper hinge: 75th percentile

Median

Lower hinge: 25th percentile

Whisker

Frequency polygon

- Construction entails drawing lines joining the mid-points of the tops of the bars of a histogram, i.e. the class mid-points. It is thus a combination of straight lines joining the frequencies at the central point in each class interval.
- Addition of extra classes with zero frequencies at either end of the frequency distribution provides a closed figure.
- This technique is particularly useful in the presence of a large number of potential class intervals.

- Frequency polygons can be superimposed upon each other, allowing comparison of two or more sets of values.

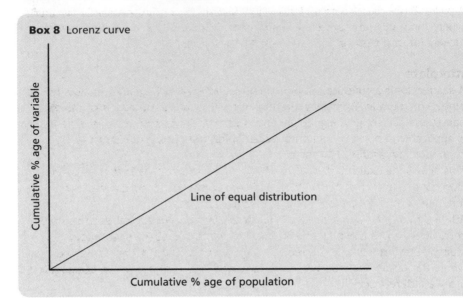

Box 8 Lorenz curve

Cumulative % age of variable (y-axis)

Line of equal distribution

Cumulative % age of population (x-axis)

Ogive
- This is a plot of the cumulative frequencies on the vertical or y axis against the upper limit of each class interval (class boundary) on the x axis. The individual data points are joined freehand.
- The cumulative frequency for a class is the total number of all observations in that class and in the previous classes. Any data point thus represents the number of observations lower in value directly below that point on a horizontal axis.
- The curve stays level or increases from left to right, often demonstrating an S-shape.

Lorenz curve
The Lorenz curve is usually used by economists to depict divergence from the average, as a measure of distribution of wealth. It has been used in health economics studies.

- It plots the cumulative percentages of the variable and of the population possessing the variable on the two axes of the same graph.
- Cumulation is always carried out in ascending order of the variable.
- The more the curve diverges from the line of equal distribution (45 degrees line), the more unequal is the actual distribution of the variable in question.
- It is useful for making comparisons of relative degrees of inequality.

Picket fence plot
- A picket is a vertical line whose length is proportional to the magnitude of the value of a variable.
- A picket fence plot is a compilation of pickets in descending order of magnitude, where the y axis represents the values of the data, and the x axis the number of pickets (or subjects), or their percentage distribution.

Scatterplots
- A scatterplot is a collection of points representing sets of x,y co-ordinates as plotted on a graph. Each set represents the values of the members of the data pair from each subject, e.g. height and weight of the same individual. The design is applicable to bivariate quantitative variables, both being measured on continuous measurement scales.
- This allows the examination of trends, linearity or curvature in the relationship, clustering of one or both variables, changes in spread of one variable as a function of the other, and the demonstration of outliers.
- A line running through the points that slopes downwards indicates a negative correlation, and a line that slopes upwards indicates a positive correlation.
- Multiple scatterplots can be used to compare observations from two studies, where the same variables have been recorded, with each group being displayed using a different scale.

Data collection

Types of statistics
- Primary: collected by the investigator.
- Secondary: obtained by the investigator from other sources and originally collected for another reason.

Methods of data collection:
- Direct observation.
- Face to face interviews.
- Postal questionnaire.
- Telephone interviews.

Modes of administration of interviews

Self administered
- Interviewer bias is avoided.
- Some questions may not be understood and may not be answered.
- Low response rate.

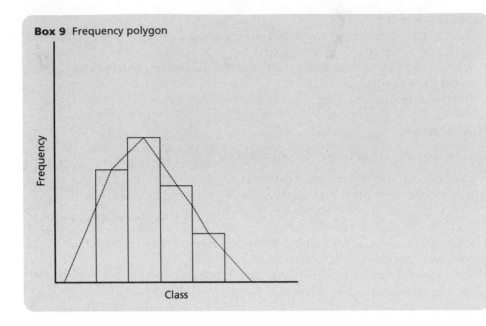

Box 9 Frequency polygon

Interviewer administered
- All questions answered.
- Allows complex questions.
- May be affected by interviewer bias.
- Cost more.

Interview types
- Informal.
- Informal but guided (semi-structured).
- Structured, with open-ended replies.
- Fully structured, with a set of possible responses for each of a fixed set of questions.

Types of questions

Recommended
- Closed-ended:
  Yes/no response
  Scaled response
  Multiple choice
  Ranking of items on question list
  Grid
  Tick boxes.
- Open-ended.
- Filter: where the respondent is directed into various streams via different options.

Not recommended
- Leading: where the question indicates the required response, increasing the probability of obtaining this response.
- Multiple: requiring more than one response from the same question, such as double-barrelled questions.
- Ambiguous or unclear.
- Loaded.
- Use of jargon.

Closed-ended questions have the following advantages:

- Standard and relatively complete answers.
- The answers are easier to code and analyse.

In general, they are preferable over open-ended questions, which may lead to:

- The collection of extensive, possibly irrelevant, information.
- Non-standard responses.
- Difficulties in coding, with low inter-coder reliability.
- Longer questionnaires.

Sampling methods

Simple random sampling
Every individual in the target population has an equal chance of inclusion in the sample data. Selection in the sample is decided by allocation based on a random sequence of numbers, i.e. a sequence with no detectable pattern. Randomisation can be achieved by tossing a coin, throwing dies, from random number tables, or by computer-generated random numbers. The latter are actually pseudo-random numbers, being generated by a deterministic algorithm, a systematic and reproducible pattern resulting whereby all sequences starting at the same point produce the same sequence of values.

Randomisation minimises bias and confounding. Bias is defined as a property of a statistic whereby its long-range average is not equal to the parameter it estimates. With bias there is a consistent and repeated divergence of the sample statistic from the population parameter in the same direction. Stated otherwise, bias is a type of systematic error that either underestimates or overestimates the inferred values of the population from the sample under study. A random sample will provide an unbiased estimate of the mean.

Systematic random sampling
Every nth item on a list is selected, the first sample unit being selected randomly, to achieve maximum dispersion over the population of size N. A convenient value for n is one which approximates N/n.

The sample frequency may correspond with a natural cycle (periodicity) in the population, leading to bias. However, the sample is spread more evenly over the entire population.

Multi-stage sampling
Frequent subdivision of the population on a random basis.

Stratified random sampling
This requires a detailed knowledge of the population under study.

The sampling frame is divided into a number of non-overlapping subpopulations or strata (e.g. ethnic groups, age groups, geographical locations, income, social class) that reflect the population make-up. Strata are chosen to be internally homogeneous, with similar values for a confounder, improving the precision of the estimate.

A separate simple random sample is obtained from each subpopulation. These are combined to make the complete sample.

Stratification can be performed on two or more variables simultaneously. In proportional allocation, the sizes of individual samples are directly proportional to the sizes of the respective strata they are drawn from.

Quota sampling
The population is stratified or broken up into different groups. The investigators are given fixed numbers (quotas) for each group targeted. They may, however, not use random methods of selecting their subjects.

Opportunity or convenience sampling
The investigator uses whatever subjects are conveniently available. In general, the use of subjects willing to participate in a trial leads to significant selection bias, rendering the results of the study unreliable.

Cluster sampling
This involves selection of a random sample of natural groups or clusters within a population, e.g. patients in a general practice or pupils in a school, and studying all subjects within each sample. Clusters are often homogeneous, relative to the population, for the variables being studied.

Utilisation of the technique is associated with loss of statistical power. There is a reduction in effective sample size caused by correlation between the subjects within clusters with respect to the outcome factor. The sample size requires multiplication by an inflation factor to satisfy the power requirements.

An intraclass or interclass correlation coefficient is required for study subjects within clusters as an estimate of the effect of clustering.

Cluster sampling saves in both time and money.

Sampling can be done either with replacement or without replacement.

With replacement
- Each member of the population may be chosen more than once.
- A finite population from which sampling is made with replacement can be considered to be infinite, i.e. unrestricted sampling is possible.

Without replacement
- Each member of the population cannot be chosen more than once.
- This is a more accurate sampling technique.

Sampling errors may be:

Random

or

Non-random
This is due to improper sampling:
- Biased sampling method, e.g. convenience sampling (selecting the easily accessible units of the population), leading to overrepresentation of one category in the sample.
- A sampling frame which differs systematically from the population, e.g. telephone directories, volunteer subjects.

The **runs test** for randomness can be used to test the hypothesis that a given data set constitutes a random sample. If the observed number of runs of data in a data set is either too large or too small to be explained by chance alone, the data set is not a random sample.

A run is a sequence of identical numbers, symbols, objects or events, preceded and followed by different numbers, symbols, objects or events, or by nothing at all.

Clinical scales
Clinical scales have a widespread use in health services research to help determine the effectiveness of therapeutic interventions. They have been devised in order to allow the standardised measurement of abstract variables, such as disability, quality of life and depression. These abstract variables are known as theoretical constructs or latent variables, and they can be defined in terms of observed empirical indicators known as constructs. This allows more objective comparison between treatments than might otherwise be possible.

Clinical scales can be based around measuring either single items, as in visual analogue scores, or measuring multiple items that are designed to define the construct under study. Scaling models are used to combine multiple items into scales. Examples of such models include summated rating scales or Likert scales. These are multi-item scales where each item is scored independently and the individual unweighted scores are summed to obtain the total score. The Barthel Index of activities of daily living is a widely used score.

The reliability of scales is measured by internal consistency and by reproducibility.

Internal consistency, or the reliability of individual items in the scale as a measure of the construct, can be determined by Cronbach's alpha or by Kuder and Richardson's formula 20.

Reproducibility refers to the agreement between two or more ratings on the same person, and can be subdivided as test-retest reliability (agreement between two or more self-report ratings for the same subject) or repeatability, intrarater reliability (agreement between two or more ratings for the same subject made by the same observer), and interrater reliability (agreement between two or more ratings for the same subject made by different observers) or observer variation. Reproducibility is reported as kappa coefficients for dichotomous data, and as intraclass correlation coefficients for continuous data (see Chapter 4).

Cronbach's alpha

This is a measure of reliability or internal consistency in a rating scale, based on the interrelation of items in the scale. It is related to both the average inter-item correlation and to the number of items in the scale (increasing as the number of items increases).

- It can take values ranging from 0 to 1.
- If there is no correlation between the items in a scale, $\alpha = 0$.
- If the items are identical and perfectly correlated, $\alpha = 1$.

Frequency distributions

A frequency distribution is a listing of all the classes or categories of a data set and the number of observations contained within each class. This represents the relation between a set of mutually exclusive and exhaustive measurement classes and the frequency of each. It depicts the number of times each value of a variable occurs in a sample or population, i.e. the frequency of occurrence of these values. An empirical frequency distribution is based on the observed data. The theoretical probability distribution is derived from a mathematical model.

The distribution of a variable can be graphically represented in several shapes, such as bell-shaped, U shaped, J or reverse J shaped, L shaped, or bimodal, which are predictive of the properties of the data they describe.

Box 10 An example of a frequency distribution can be provided from the following variates b,c,c,d,x,x,x,y as:

Variable	Frequency
b	1
c	2
d	1
x	3
y	1

Discrete probability distributions
- Binomial distribution.
- Poisson distribution.
- Hypergeometric distribution.
- Negative binomial distribution.
- Geometric distribution.
- Beta-binomial distribution.

Continuous probability distributions
- Normal distribution.
- Lognormal distribution.

- *F* distribution.
- *t* distribution.
- Chi-square distribution.
- Gamma distribution.
- Beta distribution.
- Weibull distribution.
- Logistic distribution.
- Exponential distribution.

Sampling distributions

- *t* distribution.
- Sampling distribution of sample means.

Parameters of a distribution (moments)

A distribution can be characterised by:

- The measure of central tendency.
- The measure of variability or spread.
- Skewness.
- Kurtosis.
- Modality.

Measures that characterise a distribution, e.g. measures of location and scale, are said to be robust if small changes in the distribution have a relatively small effect on their value.

A central moment is the arithmetic mean of the deviations of all items from the mrsn, each raised to the power r. The first central moment is always equal to zero. The second central moment is the variance.

Measures of the shape of a frequency curve

Skewness

The measure of the degree by which the sample population deviates from symmetry with the mean at the centre, i.e. of its symmetry.

Direction of skew: negative/positive

- Data with a long left tail is left, or negatively, skewed.
- Data with a long right tail is right, or positively, skewed.
- With a positively skewed distribution, mean > median > mode.
- With a negatively skewed distribution, mode > median > mean.

Magnitude of skew:

- Pearson's coefficient of skewness = $\dfrac{\text{mean} - \text{mode}}{\text{standard deviation}}$

  Mean − mode = 3 (mean − median).
- The sign of the number indicates direction of the skew.
- It is a pure number and has a value of zero for symmetrical distributions.

Kurtosis
Degree of peakedness or flatness of a distribution.

- Leptokurtosis: long tail.
- Platykurtosis: short tail.

The normal distribution has a kurtosis of zero.

Probability density function
The probability distribution function is a statement that specifies the upper and lower extremes of the possible values that a continuous random variable may take. It can be represented diagrammatically by a density curve, which describes the overall pattern of the frequency distribution. It is always on or above the horizontal axis.

The equation of the curve $f(x)$ is the mathematical statement that the probability density function denotes the height of the curve at the point corresponding to the chosen value of x. The probability that a random variable lies within a given interval is equal to the area under the probability distribution function corresponding to that interval.

The total area under the curve is 1.

Choice of distributions for modelling data

Discrete data
- Symmetrical: binomial distribution.
- Skewed: Poisson distribution.

Continuous data
- Symmetrical: normal distribution.
- Skewed: exponential distribution.

Binomial distribution
This is a probability distribution for discrete data with only two mutually exclusive possibilities, i.e. binary or dichotomous variables, described as success or failure. Examples of such data include alive/dead, cured/not cured, clinical sign present/absent, male/female, etc. It can also be used as a model for sampling with replacement from a finite population of any size, and as a model for sampling without replacement if the population is large in size or infinite.
A discrete random variable has a binomial distribution if:

1. There are a fixed number of trials, n.
2. Each trial can result in one of only mutually exclusive two outcomes, referred to as success or failure.
3. The probability of success in a single trial, p, is constant.
4. The trials are independent, so that the probability of success in any one trial is unaffected by the results of previous trials.

Binomial random variables are characterised by two parameters, the number of independent trials, and the probability of success per trial.

The coefficients in the formula for determining the binomial probability of r successes in n trials (i.e. the numbers pre-multiplying the x, y terms) can be obtained from **Pascal's triangle**. This is a triangle in which each new number is derived by adding the two adjacent numbers on the line above. The coefficients for n trials can be found in the appropriate line corresponding to the value of n.

The binomial distribution comprises a family of distributions, the members of which are defined by the values of n and p.

The distribution is used to model cumulative incidence rates and prevalence rates.

> **Box 11** The probability of r successes in n independent trials, given a probability of success for each trial of p, is:
>
> $$Pr = \binom{n}{r} p^r (1-p)^{n-r}$$
>
> where:
> p = probability of success in a single trial,
> $q = 1 - p$ = probability of failure
> n = number of trials, r = number of successes in n trials, $n - r$ = number of failures in n trials.
>
> $$\binom{n}{r} = \frac{n!}{r!(n-r)!}$$
>
>   = the number of ways to obtain r successes in n trials
> $n! = 1 \times 2 \times 3 \times \ldots n$
> The probabilities $p(r)$, or successive values of the probability function, are the successive terms of the binomial expansion $(q + p)^n$

Properties
- Mean = np.
- Variance = npq.
- Standard deviation = square root of ($np(1 - p)$) or square root of npq.
- Moment coefficient of kurtosis.
- Moment coefficient of skewness.

Bernoulli's theorem
If the probability of occurrence of the event X is $p(X)$, and if N trials are made, independently and under exactly the same conditions, then the probability that the relative frequency of occurrence of X differs from $p(X)$ by any amount, however small, approaches zero as the number of trials grows indefinitely large.

Poisson distribution
This is a frequency distribution for discontinuous (i.e. discrete) data or counts. These may be obtained by observing the number of discrete events in a fixed time interval or in a fixed area, length or volume.

The following requirements are necessary:

1. Events occur randomly and infrequently in a continuum such as space, time, length or volume.
2. The events are independent (there is no memory). The number of events occurring in one time interval is independent of the number occurring in previous time periods.
3. Two or more events cannot occur simultaneously. There is a small likelihood that two or more events will occur in a short time interval.

4. The mean number of events per given unit of time or space is constant. The events occur at a constant average rate
5. The expected number of events in a given interval is directly proportional to the size of the interval over which they will be counted.
6. The intervals between events, the waiting times, have an exponential distribution. If x has a Poisson distribution, $1/x$ has an exponential distribution.

Features
- The variable is the number of events that occur in an interval of given size.
- Theoretically, an infinite number of occurrences of the event must be possible in the interval.
- The distribution is completely defined by one parameter, its mean.
- The mean and variance are identical.
- The distribution is highly skewed when the mean is small.
- It tends towards normality as the mean increases.

The random variable that is equal to the distance between successive counts of a Poisson process with a mean $\lambda > 0$ has an exponential distribution with the parameter λ. An exponential random variable lacks the memory property, i.e. the probability of occurrence of an event is unrelated to any previous occurrences of the event.

> **Box 12** The probability of x random events per unit time or space is given by the formula
>
> $$P(x) = \frac{e^{-\mu} \mu^x}{x!}$$
>
> where $e = 2.71828$ (base of the natural logarithm), μ = the mean number of events in unit time or space, $x!$ = factorial x

The Poisson distribution is applicable when the probability of an individual success p becomes very small and the number of trials n becomes very large, but np (the mean) stays reasonably constant.

The Poisson distribution approximates closer to the binomial distribution as p gets smaller and n gets larger.

The distribution is used in quality control, risk analysis, the study of rare events (e.g. new cases of certain diseases, deaths from certain causes, occurrence of road traffic accidents at selected sites) and in queuing theory.

Hypergeometric distribution

The hypergeometric probability function is used to compute the probability that in a small random sample of n items out of a finite population of N items, selected without replacement, x items will be obtained labelled success and $n - x$ items labelled failure. The probability of success changes from trial to trial, and depends only on the composition of the population at the time each item is selected. In this situation the binomial distribution cannot be used as the items are not independent. This is because in a small or finite population, if one takes repeated samples without replacement, the population constantly reduces in size and its composition changes. The assumptions are:

- The population to be sampled is a finite collection of N items.
- Each individual can be characterised as either a success or a failure, being represented as a binary variable taking on the values of either 0 or 1.
- There are x successes and $n - x$ failures in the population.
- A sample of n individuals is obtained such that each subset of size n is equally likely to be chosen.

> **Box 13** Properties of hypergeometric distribution
>
> The mean $= \dfrac{n(x)}{N}$
>
> The variance $= \dfrac{n\,(x)}{(N)} \times \dfrac{(1-x)}{N} \times \dfrac{(N-n)}{(N-1)}$

Negative binomial distribution

The assumptions are:

- The experiment consists of a sequence of independent trials.
- Each trial can result in either success or failure.
- The probability of success is constant from trial to trial.
- The trials continue until a total of r successes have been observed, where r is a specified positive integer.
- The random variable of interest is x, the number of failures that precede the rth success.

The distribution can be used to describe aggregated data.

Geometric distribution

Every probability is a constant multiple of the preceding probability. The probabilities form a geometric series where each term is a constant multiple of the preceding term. This specifies probabilities for the number of trials that will be required to observe the next success.

The assumptions are:

- It comprises a sequence of trials.
- The trials are independent.
- There are only two possible outcomes at each trial.
- There is a constant probability of success at each trial.
- The variable is the number of trials taken for the first success to appear.

Normal distribution

The symmetrical bell-shaped normal curve was discovered in 1733 by Abraham de Moivre.

This provides an empirical model for many continuously distributed physiological variables, including height, weight, blood pressure, body temperature and circulating hormone levels, which tend to cluster around a central value and approximate to a normal distribution. For most physiological variables, the distribution, however, tends to be smooth, unimodal and skewed, and the mean ±2 standard deviations does not include 95% of the values.

The normal distribution is important because:

- The sampling distribution of non-normally distributed random variables tends to be normal.
- Repeated physical or physiological measurements are usually normally distributed.
- A binomial distribution that is not skewed is approximately normally distributed.
- A Poisson distribution with parameter λ can be approximated by a normal distribution when λ is large (i.e. a large mean).
- Any linear combination of independent normal random variables will have a normal distribution.

The normal distribution comprises a family of curves. Each curve is a bell-shaped curve in which the horizontal axis represents all possible values of a variable and the vertical axis the probability of those values occurring.

It is fully described by its two parameters, the mean and the variance

It is a suitable model for a variate which is continuous, unimodal and has a symmetrical frequency distribution.

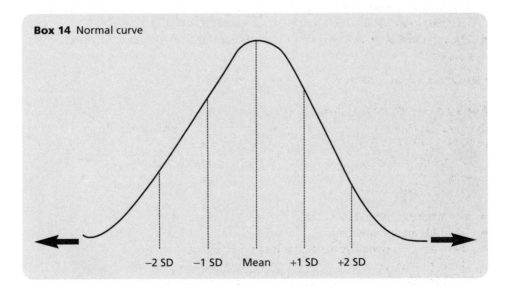

Box 14 Normal curve

−2 SD −1 SD Mean +1 SD +2 SD

Characteristics
- The mean, mode and median are equal.
- The total area under the curve is 1.
- The tails of the curve extend indefinitely in both directions, continually approaching but never touching the horizontal axis, i.e. the tails are asymptotic to the horizontal axis.
- The shape of the curve is determined by the population standard deviation.

- Distributions with small standard deviations have narrow, peaked curves and those with large standard deviations have flatter curves with less pronounced peaks.
- 68.26% of all values fall within the range of ± 1 standard deviation of the mean.
- 95.44% of all values fall within the range of ± 2 standard deviations of the mean.
- 99.73% of all values fall within the range of ± 3 standard deviations of the mean.

The reference range for a variable that defines a healthy population is taken as being equal to the mean ± 2 (strictly 1.96) standard deviations (parametric 95% range).

This range is defined by the 95 percentile range, bounded by the 2.5th and 97.5th percentiles, of the empirical distribution of the observations if they are not normally distributed.

Properties
- Mean.
- Variance.
- Standard deviation.
- Moment coefficient of skewness.
- Moment coefficient of kurtosis.
- Mean deviation.

Standard normal distribution (Z distribution)

This is a normal distribution with a mean of 0, a standard deviation of 1 and a variance of 1. It is a reference distribution from which information about other normal distributions can be obtained. The use of this distribution lies in the fact that a single table may be employed for the areas of the normal curve by the utilisation of standard deviation units.

Observations from a normal distribution are often expressed in standard deviation units about the mean based on this Z distribution. This is called a Z score, which is equal to the observed score – population mean/population standard deviation. The Z score is dimensionless. A positive Z score indicates that the observation is greater than the mean. A negative Z score indicates that the observation is less than the mean.

The requisites for a Z test are:

- Random samples.
- Quantitative data.
- Variable normally distributed in the population.
- Sample size greater than 30.

Normal area tables show the area under the normal curve between the mean and any given number of standard deviations.

Tables that detail the standard normal distribution can be used for transformed data from any normal distribution. A standard measure of the distance of the score from the mean is obtained. A standardised score shows the relative location of that score in the frequency distribution.

To transform to the standard normal distribution:

- Subtract the mean from each x value.
- Divide the remainders by the standard deviation.

This represents a linear transformation, which retains the underlying relationship among the values of the parent normal distribution.

Central limit theorem (de Moivre)

The central limit theorem specifies the nature of the sampling distribution of the mean. This is a frequency distribution of a large number of sample means of size n that are drawn from a given population.

The theorem states that, for an infinite number of independent random samples of equal size selected from a population, the sampling distribution of any linear combination of the sample means will approach a normal distribution as the size of each sample approaches infinity. That is, as sample size n increases, the sampling distribution approaches a normal distribution.

If a series of samples is drawn from a population and the mean of the observations calculated in each sample, the means comprise a set. The set of sample means always form a normal distribution irrespective of whether or not they were drawn from a normally distributed population. The sample means are normally distributed around the population mean.

The standard deviation of the set of means, the standard error of means, is equal to the population standard deviation/square root of the sample size. 95% of sample means will lie within 2 standard errors of the population mean as long as n, the sample size, is greater than 30. The standard error is in the same units as the standard deviation, and is the best estimate of the sampling error.

Regardless of the shape of the distribution of a population, the normal distribution can be applied provided that the sample is representative and the sample size is equal to or greater than 30. Sample size must not be confused with the number of samples. The greater the heterogeneity (as measured by the standard deviation) of the sample, the larger the sample size must be in order for the sample mean to be an accurate estimate of the population mean.

Testing sample data for normality

- Plotting data in the form of a histogram shows a unimodal distribution.
- Stem and leaf plot and box plot procedures to detect outliers and unusual data structure.
- Normal probability or probit plot.

  Transform measured values into standard normal deviate values (normal scores) by subtracting the mean and dividing by the standard deviation, and then rank them in ascending order.

A plot of the cumulative ranked scores from a true normal distribution with a mean of zero and a standard deviation of 1 on the y axis against the measured values (the sample data) on the x axis gives a perfect straight line. It is a comparison of the cumulative frequency distributions of the data against that of the standard normal deviation.

- Examination of the coefficients of skewness and kurtosis.
- Shapiro–Wilk W test: a ratio of estimates of the variance.
- Kolmogorov–Smirnov test or the Lilliefor's modification.
- Chi-square test: based on the deviations between a data histogram and the theoretical density function.

Kolmogorov–Smirnov one-sample test

The test is a test of goodness-of-fit for variables, which are measured on at least an ordinal scale, based on the deviations between the empirical probability distribution and the theoretical distribution function. The variables should represent random samples from a continuous theoretical distribution, the sample size not being important.

It determines whether the scores in a sample can be thought to have come from a population having a specified theoretical distribution.

It is a non-parametric test of the null hypothesis that two cumulative frequency distributions are the same. The value of the statistic is the maximum absolute difference between the two empirical cumulative distribution functions. The Lilliefor's modification tests the null hypothesis of normality.

Kolmogorov–Smirnov two-sample test

This a test of whether two independent samples have been drawn from the same population or from populations with the same distribution.

The two-tailed test is sensitive to any kind of difference in the distributions from which the two samples were drawn (i.e. in central tendency, dispersion, skewness, etc.). The one-tailed test is used to decide whether or not the data values in the population from which one of the samples are drawn is stochastically larger than the values of the population from which the other sample was drawn.

Lognormal distribution

This represents a random variable whose logarithm follows a normal distribution. It is applicable to random variables that are constrained by zero but have a few very large values. The distribution is asymmetrical and positively skewed, with a greater probability in the right tail.

F distribution

A family of distributions characterised by two parameters, degrees of freedom for the numerator and degrees of freedom for the denominator, i.e. the degrees of freedom for the estimates of variance in random samples from normal distributions with the same variance.

Features

- The numerator has $(I - 1)$ degrees of freedom, where I is the number of populations being compared.
- The denominator has $(N - I)$ degrees of freedom, where $N =$ total number of observations.

- The sampling within the sets should be random.
- Variances from within the various sets must be approximately equal.
- Observations within the experimentally homogeneous sets should be from normally distributed populations.
- Contributions to total variance must be additive.
- The shape in general is skewed to the right, i.e. positively skewed.
- A random variable that has an F distribution cannot assume a negative value.

t distribution

The t distribution was first described by William Sealy Gossett ('Student'), a brewer with Arthur Guinness and Company at St James's Gate, Dublin.

Features
- A bell shaped distribution, which describes the variability of the mean and standard deviation of small samples taken from a normally distributed population.
- It has a lower height and a wider spread (i.e. larger standard deviation) than a standard normal deviation.
- A t random variable has a higher chance of being further from the mean than a standard normal random variable. The critical values of t for a specified level of significance are larger than the corresponding critical values for z.
- It comprises a family of distributions of sample means, each characterised by its degrees of freedom (df $= N - 1$).
- The smaller the degrees of freedom, the flatter the shape of the distribution, resulting in a greater area in the tails of the distribution.
- It closely approximates a standard normal distribution for sample sizes of 60 or over.
- The variance approaches 1 as the sample size becomes large.

Chi-square distribution

Features
- A family of probability distributions, each characterised by its degrees of freedom.
- The distribution results when repeated random samples of n independent values of a normally distributed variable x are obtained, each x value is transformed to the standard normal distribution, and the results are squared and summed.
- The mean is equal to the degrees of freedom.
- The variance is equal to 2 × degrees of freedom, i.e. 2 × mean.
- The mode is at mean − 2 for mean $\geqq 2$.
- Chi-square takes on values between zero and (positive) infinity.
- The distribution has a long right hand tail and is highly skewed to the right. The function approaches the chi-square axis asymptotically only at the right hand tail.
- The distribution becomes more symmetrical or bell shaped as the degrees of freedom increase.
- The total area under the curve is equal to 1.

Weibull distribution

The two-parameter Weibull distribution can represent decreasing, constant or increasing failure rates. The distribution is used to model time until failure of many different physical systems, and has been extended to survival analysis in biological systems. The distribution allows extrapolation from high to low dose exposures, e.g. from occupational to environmental.

Exponential distribution

This models events recurring randomly over time. This is the only continuous distribution that is memory-less (with no memory of where or when it started, the current time having no effect on future outcomes) and the only continuous distribution with a constant hazard function. It has no shape or location parameters.

Chebyshev's theorem or inequality

Given a set of n observations $x_1, x_2, x_3, \ldots x_n$ on a variable X, the probability is at least $(1 - -1/k^2)$ that X will take on a value within k (where k is greater than 1) standard deviations of the mean of the set of observations.

The probability that a random variable X will differ absolutely from expectation by b or more units ($b > 0$) is always less than, or equal to, the ratio of the variance to b^2. This allows the use of the mean and standard deviation of any set of data to categorise the whole group.

Chebyshev's theorem is true for all probability distributions and can be applied to any data set, regardless of the shape of the frequency distribution of the data.

Sampling distribution

A sampling distribution is a theoretical probability distribution that relates the possible values of a statistic based on a sample of N cases, and the probability (density) associated with each value.

The sampling distribution of the mean is the theoretical probability distribution relating the possible values of the sample mean to the probability (density) of each.

Data transformations

A transformation applied to a variable changes each value of the variable as described by the transformation.

Transformations are useful in the following circumstances:

- When a continuous variable does not follow a normal distribution, the data can be transformed into a normal distribution. This reduces the degree of skewness and allows the use of parametric statistical testing.
- Where variance over the range of the data in regression analysis and in analysis of variance is not constant (to stabilise variance).
- To linearise relationships among paired data sets, such as may occur when fitting a least squares line.
- To depict data on a more convenient scale, allowing easier data manipulation.
- To reduce the effect of outliers.
- To make the effects of treatments additive.

The use of the logarithmic pH scale is an example of the use of transformed data in common usage.

Transformation of sample data to a normal distribution

Logarithmic transform

The logarithm of a base number is the power to which 10 or e (an irrational number with a value of 2.7182818) should be raised to obtain it. A logarithmic transformation changes multiplicative behaviour into additive behaviour, division into subtraction, and exponential behaviour into multiplicative.

The logarithmic scale is useful for the transformation of positively skewed distributions. The scale is characterised by the fact that the ratio between equidistant points is equal.

The transformation is appropriate when the variances are proportional to the square of means. The logarithmic scale is useful when the variable under study has a large standard deviation compared to its mean. Logarithmic transformations are used in studies related to the growth of organisms.

> **Box 15** Logarithmic transformation
>
> Transform xi to $yi = \log a(x_i)$ where a is 10. $\log e(x_i)$ may be used to obtain the same overall effect, the only difference being the numerical scaling of y.

The lognormal distribution can be transformed to a normal distribution by taking the natural logarithm of each observation. The values for the observations need to be positive.

Modified log-transform

> **Box 16** Modified logarithmic transformation
>
> $y_i = \log e(x_i + k)$
> k = an additive constant that gives a coefficient of skewness = 0 for the subsequently transformed xi values

Exponential transform

Modulus transform

Choice of methods of transformations to normality

- Data skewed to the right (positive skew):
  $1/x$ (reciprocal)
  $\log x$ (logarithmic)
  square root of x (appropriate when the variances are proportional to the means): applicable where the variable is a count with a Poisson distribution.
- Data skewed to the left (negative skew)
  x squared

x cubed(cubic)

e*x*.

Linearising a relationship

Log transformation (when standard deviation is proportional to the mean)
- The natural logarithms of the values of the variable are used.

Power transformation
- Square transformation.
- Box Cox transformations, e.g.

$$x' = \frac{v}{(x-1)} v.$$

where *v* is not equal to 0.

Logit transformation

Trigonometric transformations
- The arcsine transformation (the arcsine of a number is the angle whose sine is that number) is used to transform percentages or proportions from a binomial distribution to a nearly normal distribution.
- Each proportion is expressed as a number between 0 and 1.
- The inverse sine (arcsine) of the square root of each proportion is determined.
- Each observation is weighted by the number in the denominator of the proportion.
- Each of the original observations is thus replaced by an angle whose sine is the square root of the original observation.

Chapter 3

Correlation and regression

Correlation and regression are essentially methods to study the magnitude of the association between, and the functional relation between, two or more variables. Correlation is primarily designed to determine the interdependence of two variables, which may or may not be functionally related. It is not a predictive tool, and the simultaneous changes in two variables may be purely coincidental, as shown in a study correlating increased births in a community with increased sightings of storks.

Correlation indicates a mathematical association between two variables; this is not necessarily a cause and effect relationship.

Regression, on the other hand, determines the functional dependence of a dependent variable on one or more independent variable. This allows prediction of this dependent variable with variations in the independent variables.

Regression

Regression indicates a mathematical relationship between a dependent (or outcome or response) variable, and one or more independent (or predictor or explanatory or regressor) variables. Independent variables are manipulated and dependent variables are measured. Regression analysis is used to predict one variable from another, thereby assessing functional dependency.

The term regression to the mean (originally mediocrity!) was originated by Francis Galton, while investigating the relationship between the heights of children and of their parents in 1886. This does not strictly coincide with the context in which the term is currently used. Galton noted that tall fathers tended to have shorter sons, and short fathers to have taller sons. Thus extreme values of characteristics tend to even out in the offspring. Regression to the mean is seen with any variable that fluctuates in value within any individual, either genuinely or due to measurement error, e.g. serum levels of cholesterol.

Simple linear regression and multiple regression are appropriate for continuous response variables, e.g. blood pressure, weight.

Logistic regression is applicable to situations involving binary response variables, e.g. dead/alive, recovered/not recovered (i.e., the response of interest is a dichotomous random variable).A logistic model is a linear model on the logit scale. The logit of the outcome is modelled as the sum of the individual independent variables.

Measures of the relationship between two interval/ratio-measured variables

1. Parametric:
   (i)   Pearson's product moment correlation coefficient.
2. Non-parametric:
   (i)   Spearman's rank-order correlation coefficient
   (ii)   Kendall's tau.

Pearson's product moment correlation coefficient

This is a measure of the strength of relationship between interval/ratio variables. It has no predictive value. It requires that:

- Both variables are continuous, and at least one follows a normal distribution.
- The relationship is linear.
- The sample is of adequate size to assume normality.

Pearson's correlation coefficient, r, can be calculated from the gradients of the two regression lines

---

Box 17 Calculation of Pearson's r

$r = m/M$

m = gradient from regression equation $y = mx + c$; M = gradient from regression equation $x = 1/My + c$

It can thereby be regarded as a measure of scatter around the regression line. With no correlation ($r = 0$), there is maximum scatter around the regression line.
   The correlation coefficient is usually obtained from the formula

$$r = \frac{SSxy}{\sqrt{SSxx\ SSyy}}$$

or

$$\frac{\text{sum of the product of the deviations of the means of } x \text{ and } y \text{ values}}{\text{sum of the product of the standard deviations}}$$

where: m measurements are made on variables x and y,
SS = sum of squares

$$SSxy = \Sigma xy - \frac{(\Sigma x)(\Sigma y)}{n}$$

$$SSxx = \Sigma x^2 - \frac{(\Sigma x)^2}{n}$$

$$SSyy = \Sigma y^2 - \frac{(\Sigma y)^2}{n}$$

Properties
- r can assume values from −1 (perfect negative relationship) to +1 (perfect positive relationship), inclusive.
- r is positive for direct relationships, i.e. as one variable increases so does the other.
- r is negative for indirect relationships, i.e. as one variable increases the other decreases.
- The sign of r is equal to the sign of the slope of the regression line.
- A correlation of 0 (independence) indicates the lack of a linear relationship between the two variables.
- There are no units for measurement.
- The value is independent of the units to measure the variables.
- The value can be markedly affected by an outlier, hence it is not suitable for use with skewed distributions.
- When testing hypotheses relating to the correlation coefficient, effect size is estimated as the smallest value of the coefficient that can be detected.

A positive correlation may occur between two variables x and y when:

- x causes y.
- y causes x.
- Another variable causes both x and y.
- There is a spurious association between x and y.

Potential fallacies of calculated correlation coefficients
- Correlation does not imply a cause-and-effect relationship. High correlation may turn out to be nonsensical.
- Correlation is a measure of association or linear relation only.
- It can be misleading from the influence of a third variable.

Thus two variables may be highly correlated because either X causes Y, Y causes X, or both X and Y are caused by some third variable.

- It is highly sensitive to outliers.
- Inferences may be made to an unsampled population.

Spearman's rank correlation coefficient (Spearman's rho)

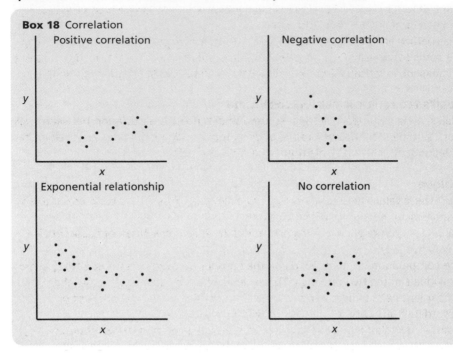

Box 18 Correlation

Positive correlation

Negative correlation

Exponential relationship

No correlation

Requirements
- Uses non-parametric data, i.e. ranks rather than the actual observations.
- The variables are measured on at least an ordinal scale. Individual observations can be ranked into two ordered series.
- Both variables are continuous.
- No assumption is made about the distribution of either variable.
- The relationship between the two variables is monotonic.

Technique
- Rank x values among themselves, assigning rank 1 to smallest (or largest) value, rank 2 to the second smallest (or largest) value, and so on.
- Rank y values similarly among themselves.
- The ranks in the same row must be for the same observation.
- Find the sum of the squares of the differences, d, between the ranks of x values and corresponding y values: Σd^2.
- Substitute into the formula

$$r = 1 - \frac{6(\Sigma d)^2}{n(n^2 - 1)}$$

Where n = number of pairs of observations
- When there are ties in ranks, assign to each of the tied observations the arithmetic mean of the ranks which they jointly occupy.

- If there are too many ties, a correction factor is needed.
- The null hypothesis is that there is no significant correlation between the sets of x and y values, i.e. the value of r is 0.
- The coefficient may range from -1 to $+1$. $+1$ indicates perfect agreement between the ranks of the values, i.e. all pairs of ranks are identical. -1 indicates that no pairs of ranks are identical. 0 indicates that there is no pattern to the pairs of ranks.

Kendall's tau rank correlation coefficient
Kendall's tau is a non-parametric test, used to describe the association between two random variables, either two ordinal or one ordinal and one continuous variable, in an independent, identically distributed sample of n pairs.

Technique
- Rank the x values and the y values in two separate rows. The n pairs are ordered in increasing magnitude of the x values.
- If x and y are independent, any of the $n!$ orderings of the ranks of the y variable is equally likely.
- The computation of tau depends on the number of inversions in order for pairs of individuals in the two rankings. This is determined by counting the number of concordant pairs (where y increases with increasing x) and the number of discordant pairs (where y decreases with increasing x).
- A single inversion in order exists between any pairs of individuals when one is greater than the other in one ranking and the other greater in the second ranking. When the two rankings are identical (tied pairs), no inversions in order exist. When one ranking is exactly the reverse of the other, an inversion exists for each pair of individuals.
- An inversion in order for any pair of objects is treated in the same way as evidence for disagreement.
- In the presence of positive correlation, the y values will tend to increase, more often than to decrease, as x increases. The opposite occurs in the presence of negative correlation.
- The test statistic assumes extreme values of the x and y values are associated or correlated.
- $\tau = 1 - [2$ (number of inversions)/number of pairs of objects] or number of concordant pairs $-$ number of discordant pairs/$n(n - 1)/2$.
- There are three variants of the test, tau a, tau b and tau c, depending on usage.
- Tau will always assume a value between -1 (complete discordance) and $+1$ (complete concordance).

Linear regression analysis
Regression analysis is a technique for investigating and modelling the relationship between variables, where one variable is predictive of the other.

The aim of regression analysis is to find the best fitting and most parsimonious model to describe the relationship between a dependent (outcome or response) variable and a set of independent (predictor or explanatory) variables.

The model is based on the assumption that the relationship between the variables comprises a systematic or deterministic component represented by a straight line, and a random or stochastic component represented by the deviations of the observed data about this line.

Use of regression models

- Summarise or describe a data set, and to describe and model a relationship between the dependent variable and one or more independent variables.
- Estimate a parameter.
- Predict a dependent variable from some particular values of the independent variables.
- Test hypotheses about associations between variables comparing alternative models of association.

Method

- Scatterplots of the dependent variable (on the y axis) are plotted against each of the independent variables, either one independent variable in simple linear regression or multiple in multiple linear regression (on the x axis). Each pair of x, y observations is plotted as a single point.
- The linear (straight-line) relationship between the variables, and any deviations from linearity, is assessed by inspection of the scatterplots.
- The correlation between the independent variables is ascertained by scatterplots and correlation coefficients.
- Outliers may indicate either an error in measurement, the true value for an unusual member of the population, or observations on a subject that does not belong in the study population.
- The starting independent variables are selected.

The method of entry into the model is decided (if multiple regression). The fit of model is determined by the value for r^2 (simple linear regression) or adjusted r^2 (multiple regression), where r is the correlation coefficient and r^2 is the coefficient of determination, and by assessing the residuals. The residual represents unexplained (or residual) variation after fitting a regression model. It is the difference between the observed value of the variable and the value predicted by the regression model.

- Multicollinearity (correlation – a linear or near linear relation – among the independent variables) between the selected variables is looked for and the residuals checked for non-normality and then plotted against the predicted values.
- One should not extrapolate beyond the range of sample data. Regression models are intended as interpolation equations over the range of the independent variables used to fit the model. Regression is only valid in the range in which data are available. One cannot predict values of the predictor variable outside the range of observed values of the variable.
- If the data do not seem to lie on a line, or if the residuals show a clear pattern, the linear model may not be consistent with the data.

- If the data seem to follow a particular curve, such as a logarithmic, sinusoidal or exponential curve, non-linear regression is appropriate.
- If part of the data seem to lie along one line and part along another line, the data can be stratified, fitting a different line to each segment of the data.
- Another solution to the problem of non-linearity is transformation. The measurements of the x or y variable are changed to a different scale, such as logarithmic.

r^2, the **coefficient of determination**, is that proportion of the total variability in the dependent variable that is accounted for by the regression equation. It indicates how much of the change in y is explained by x. The value of r^2 is thus an indicator of how well the regression model fits the data. When r^2 is 1 it indicates that the fitted equation accounts for all the variability of the values of the dependent variables in the sample distribution. A value near 0 indicates poor fit.

In a bivariate normal distribution, there are always two regression lines, that of y on x, and of x on y. The correlation coefficient is the geometric mean of the slopes of these two lines.

Non-linear regression

- If plotting of paired data on semi-log paper (with equal subdivisions for x and a logarithmic scale for y) yields an approximately straight line, this indicates that an exponential curve will give a good fit for the data.
- If plotting of paired data on log–log paper (with logarithmic scales for both x, b and y) yields an approximately straight line, the equation $y = a.x^b$ will provide a good fit for the data.
- If on plotting paired data, y values initially increase and then decrease, or vice versa, given the arrangement of x values in ascending order of magnitude, a parabolic equation will give a good fit for the data, according to the equation $y = a + b1x + b2x^2$, where a is the y intercept (where the regression line crosses the y axis), and b is the slope or gradient (direction and steepness) of the line.

Least squares method

This is a method of estimating the unknown parameters in the regression model, i.e. of fitting the model to the data. The method produces the best unbiased estimators of the regression coefficients. The general method of estimation that leads to the least squares function under the linear regression model is called maximum likelihood.

Method

- This involves fitting a straight line to data consisting of paired observations of two variables x and y.
- The line fitted to the data should be such that the sum of the squares of the vertical deviations from the points to the line, i.e. the sum of the squares of the residuals, is a minimum (best fit). Positive deviations lie above the line, and negative deviations below the line.

The assumptions made include:

- The y variable is normally distributed for each value of x.
- The variability of y is the same over the range of values of x investigated.
- The values of y are independent of one another.
- The observations are a random sample from the population.
- The relationship between x and y is linear.

The least square line minimises the sum of squares of errors. As the errors are squared, the chance of negative errors cancelling positive errors is removed. The two properties of the least squares line are:

- The sum of errors, i.e. the sum of the differences of the points above and below the straight line, is equal to 0.
- The sum of squared errors is smaller than that for any other straight line model.

Assumptions underlying a simple linear regression model

- **Normality:** the deviations (scatter) of data values from the line are normally distributed.
- **Linearity:** the relation is linear. The means of the subpopulations of Y all lie on the same line.
- **Homoscedasticity:** like or equal scatter, i.e. equal vertical dispersions. All Y distributions have an identical variance, i.e. the dependent variable(s) demonstrate equal levels of variance across the range of predictor variable(s). Heteroscedasticity is revealed if the residuals tend to increase or decrease with values of the predictor variable. It can be removed by working with transformed variables.
- **Independence:** Y values are statistically independent.
- **Random sampling**

The regression line for Y on X estimates the average value of Y corresponding to each value of X. The slope of the regression line $= r \times$ standard deviation of Y/standard deviation of X.

The assumptions underlying a regression analysis can be tested by:

- Residual plots: a scatter plot of the residual against X or the fitted value.
- A normal probability plot of the residuals.
- A time-series plot of the residuals: a scatter plot of the residuals against time, which can uncover correlation between error terms over time.

The precision and accuracy of a regression analysis can be affected by:

- Random sampling errors.
- The precision of the observations for each individual sample.
- The number of observations.
- The range of values of the X variable.
- The offset of the range of X values: clustering of the X values at some offset from the origin.
- Extent of scatter about the regression.

Multiple regression

The prediction of a single dependent (or response or outcome) variable by two or more independent (or predictor, explanatory, regressor variables, or covariates) variables considered simultaneously, and determination of the extent to which each independent variable influences the dependent variable.

The dependent variable is related to the independent variable by a best fit.

Method

- **Stepwise methods** can be used to choose the best set of independent variables from a large set. This can be achieved either by forward selection or step-up (adding variables one at a time into the regression), or by backward elimination or step-down (removing one variable at a time) from a model in which all independent variables under consideration are used.
- With **forward selection methods** the order of fitting is determined by using the partial correlation coefficient as a measure of importance of variables not yet in the fitted equation. The partial correlation coefficient considers correlation between each pair of variables while maintaining constant the value of each of the other variables. At each stage, the value of adding or removing variables can be tested using variance ratio (F tests) methods.
- **Backward elimination** is more likely to detect a variable that is significant only when a suppressor variable is in the model.
- When the independent variables are highly correlated with one another (multicollinearity, or non-linear dependence among the independent variables), the model relating independent variables to the dependent variable can be seriously distorted. With extreme multicollinearity at least two of the independent variables are perfectly related by a linear function. Near-extreme multicollinearity means that there are strong (but not perfect) linear relationships among the independent variables. Forward selection is the better method with small sample sizes or in the presence of concerns about multicollinearity.
- In observational studies, the bias of some of the confounding variables can be eliminated by including them as regressors.
- The change in the mean value of the outcome is modelled as the sum of the individual effects of the independent variables on outcome.

Stepwise methods for selection or elimination of independent variables from a model are based on a statistical algorithm that checks for the importance of the variables, either including or excluding them on the basis of a fixed decision rule. The importance of a variable is defined as a measure of the statistical significance of the partial correlation coefficient for the variable. The partial correlation coefficient is the correlation of an independent and dependent variable when the effects of other independent variable(s) have been removed from both.

The more variables that are included in a model, the greater the estimated standard errors become, and the higher the dependence of the model on the observed data. Different sets of independent variables may be arrived at by the use of different stepwise techniques, whether step-up or step-down.

Multiple regression may be used to:

- Combine multiple independent variables to produce an optimal prediction of the dependent variable, or
- Separate the effects of the independent variables on the dependent variable (causal analysis). This aims to determine whether a particular independent variable affects the dependent variable, and to estimate the magnitude of the effect.
- Test for the presence of interactions, i.e. effect modifiers.

Box 19 Multiple regression equation

The relationship between a single dependent variable y and multiple independent variables x is stated by an additive equation:

$y = a + b_1x_1 + b_2x_2 + \ldots b_kx_k + \varepsilon$

where $x_1 \ldots x_k$ represent the independent variables, ε = a random error variable with a normal distribution, $a, b_1 \ldots b_k$ are the partial regression coefficients. Each of these coefficients indicates only the effect of its independent variable on the dependent variable, with the effects of all other independent variables in the equation controlled for.

Assumptions required for using multiple linear regression
- The variables are drawn from a normally distributed population of scores.
- Independent or explanatory variables are linearly related to the dependent or predictor variable (a continuous random variable). The variance of y values is the same for all values of $x_1 \ldots x_k$.
- The independent variables may be either random or non-random (fixed) variables.
- The residuals (differences between observed and estimated values) are independent.
- The residuals are normally distributed with zero mean and constant variance.
- Outliers (extreme scores) eliminated. These can be univariate (extreme score on one variable) or multivariate (extreme score on two variables together).
- Multicollinearity: The independent variables have high correlations with each other. Highly correlated variables can be combined, with reduction of the number of variables.

Coded qualitative independent variables with a restricted range of values are known as **dummy variables**. Coding is a standard method of incorporating dichotomous variables in a regression equation, coded as either 1 or 0. This allows multivariate analyses on ordinal and nominal variables.

Methods of detection of outliers in multiple linear regression models
- Graphical presentation: scatter plots.
- Standardised residuals: value > 2–3 suggest an outlier.
- Studentised residuals: values > 2–3 suggest an outlier.
- Cook's distance: a measure of the change in the regression coefficients with elimination of the outlier.

Polynomial regression is a form of multiple regression in which the independent variables are powers of the dependent variable. This allows fitting of a regression model to curvilinear relationships without the need for data transformation. The highest-degree polynomial that may be fitted to the data is one less than the number of observations.

Poisson regression

The relationship between a response variable and a potentially useful predictor variable is studied using Poisson regression when:

- The response variable is not normally distributed.
- The response variable represents a count of a relatively rare event.
- The study is large in size.

The logarithm of the rate (link function) is a linear function of the risk factors or predictor variables.

The method is applicable to multivariate analysis of factors affecting incidence of disease or death rates in cohort studies, where these outcome events are relatively rare.

Straight line equation

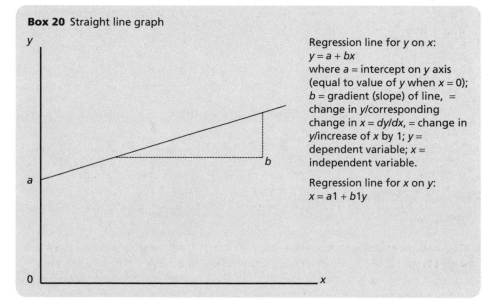

Box 20 Straight line graph

Regression line for y on x:
$y = a + bx$
where a = intercept on y axis (equal to value of y when $x = 0$); b = gradient (slope) of line, = change in y/corresponding change in $x = dy/dx$, = change in y/increase of x by 1; y = dependent variable; x = independent variable.

Regression line for x on y:
$x = a1 + b1y$

Non-linear equations

$y = a + bx^2$ (exponential curve)
or $\log y = \log a + x(\log b)$, where log is logarithm to the base 10
$y = a + b\sqrt{x}$
$y = a + b/x^2$

$$y = a + b/x$$
$$y = ax^b$$
or $\log y = \log a + b(\log x)$

Log-linear model

The traditional distinction between dependent and independent variables is dropped. All variables are entered as continuous variables. The model examines the direct and interactive relationships of all variables to each other. Goodness-of-fit statistics are computed using chi-square or likelihood-ratio chi squares.

Logistic regression

Logit models are a class of models used to explore the relationship of a binary or dichotomous categorical dependent or response variable (which takes one of two values, usually the occurrence or non-occurrence of some outcome event) to one or more independent or explanatory categorical or continuous variables. The odds ratio is used as a measure of association, the dependent variable being the log-odds. Multiple logistic regression models are used to model disease risk over a study period as a function of multiple risk factors. A classic example is the Framingham cohort study.

The logit, or **log-odds** (the natural logarithm of the odds of the outcome) that the dependent variable has a specific given value, is analysed as a linear function of the independent variables.

Logit models are analogous to regression models in which the expected value of a continuous dependent variable is expressed as linear combination/function of one or more independent variables.

The models compare the observed values of the logit transformation (log-odds) of the dependent variable to predicted values obtained from models with and without the binary variable under study.

In a multivariate logistic regression model the estimated effect of each variable in the model is adjusted for differences in the distributions of, and associations among, the other independent variables. Each estimated regression coefficient provides an estimate of the log-odds adjusting for all other variables and included in the model.

Generalised linear models

These models are used to demonstrate the linear and non-linear relationships between a discrete or continuous dependent (y) variable and a set of independent variables (x), where the responses are independent. They are extensions of linear multiple regression models in which the underlying systematic component is a specified function of a linear combination of the parameters – a linear predictor. The linear predictor connects the independent variables to the dependent variable. Model fitting is by an iterative weighted least squares algorithm.

Generalised linear models allow regression analysis where the assumptions of normality and of constant variance do not hold. The dependent variable is assumed to be obtained from a member of the exponential family of distributions, including the normal, Poisson, binomial, exponential and gamma distributions.

The assumptions are:

- There are n observations of a dependent variable y.
- Each y is composed of a systematic component and a random component.
- There is a linear predictor.
- There is a link function, which creates a linear relationship between the variable(s) under study and the dependent variable.

Classification of generalised linear models

Univariate generalised linear models
- Binary and binomial responses:
  Linear probability models
  Logit models
  Probit models
  Complementary log-log models.
- Count data:
  Log-linear Poisson models
  Linear Poisson models.

Bayesian generalised linear models

Multivariate extensions of generalised linear models
- Ordinal responses:
  Cumulative models:
    Cumulative logistic models or proportional odds models for ordered categorical data
    Grouped Cox models or proportional hazards models for survival data
    Extreme maximal-value distribution models.
  Sequential models:
  Two-step models.

Canonical correlation analysis

This is a multivariate statistical model that simultaneously correlates several quantitative dependent variables and several quantitative independent variables, seeking to obtain the maximum correlation between the two sets of variables. It thus quantifies the strength of relationship between these two sets. It is a logical extension of multiple regression. A sequence of pairs of patterns in two multivariate data sets is identified, and sets of transformed variables are constructed by projecting the original data on to these patterns. A canonical variable is a linear combination of the components of a multivariate observation, reducing the dimensionality of the observation.

Method
- Linear combinations of variables are selected from two sets of variables. A number of independent canonical functions are derived that maximise the Pearson product-moment correlations between the linear components of sets of independent and dependent variables.

- Each canonical function is based on the correlation between two canonical variates, one for dependent variables and one for independent variables.
- Sets of weights are derived for dependent and independent variables that result in the highest possible correlation between the composite variates.

Assumptions
- Independent random samples.
- Multivariate normality.
- No singularities.
- Linearity.

Recursive partitioning
This includes two classes of non-parametric regression methods, which are used to explore data structures and to derive parsimonious models from them by partitioning the subjects into subgroups with different risks of outcome. A recursive model is a one-way model, with no feedback loops.

Classification And Regression Tree (CART) technique
This is used for the prediction of continuous dependent variables (regression) and categorical predictor variables (classification).

A tree structure is generated by recursive division of the sample into a number of subgroups, using a tree-building algorithm. Each division is chosen to maximise some measure of the difference in the response variable in the resulting groups, i.e. there is sequential choice of the strongest risk factors for the outcome. Each subgroup is as homogeneous as possible with regards to the outcome. Partitioning and pruning of the tree structure allows derivation of the desired model.

CART techniques have been used in the development of decision rules, such as for identifying patients with chest pain at high risk of this being due to myocardial ischaemia, and in the derivation of radiological decision support rules such as the Ottawa Ankle Rules.

- Multivariate adaptive regression splines

Statistical testing

Hypothesis testing is one of the most important applications of statistics to medical research. This is centred around the statement of a null hypothesis, usually one to the effect that the intervention under study does not have a significant beneficial effect, and an alternative or research hypothesis. One starts out with the belief that the intervention does not work, any differences between the study groups being due to chance only, and aims to disprove this, i.e. to reject the null hypothesis. The choice of statistical test is decided primarily by the properties of the sample data and their expected distribution, as outlined below.

Choice of statistical method for data analysis

This depends on:

- The purpose of the analysis:
  Predicted change or difference, whether uni-directional or in either direction
  Predicted association.
- Type of data.
- Assumptions about the data being normally or non-normally distributed:
  Parametric tests are used when data are in the interval or ratio scale, or are normally distributed.
- Study design:
  Paired data (repeated measurements on the same subjects, and matched case-control comparisons)
  Independent data.
- Number of groups.

Non-parametric tests are used when:

- Data are in nominal or ordinal scales. Order or rank may be used in place of the numerical values of the observations.
- No estimates of parameters (e.g. mean or standard deviation) or distributional assumptions (assumptions about the underlying populations from which the data are obtained) are necessary.
- Interval, continuous or ratio scale data deviate markedly from normality.
- Sample sizes are small – this is an incorrect application. Note that non-parametric tests lack statistical power with small samples.

However:

- Statistical power is smaller than for the analogous parametric test.
- type II error is more likely.
- Larger sample sizes are needed to detect differences between means.
- Confidence intervals cannot be readily provided.

Non-parametric tests are relatively insensitive to outliers.

Designs

- With related designs (same or matched subjects) the differences between subjects' scores under different experimental conditions are rank ordered. Tied ranks based on average ranks are allocated to identical differences between scores. Positive and negative differences are ranked together.
- With unrelated designs (different subjects) all scores are pooled and rank ordered to calculate overall differences between different experimental conditions. Identical scores are allocated tied ranks, calculated on the basis of the average of the ranks, which should have been allocated to these scores.

Parametric tests are used when:

- Data are in at least an interval scale.
- The sample data are drawn from a normally distributed population.
- The variances of the two samples are not significantly different, i.e. there is homogeneity of variance.

Sample size calculation

The size of the sample depends on:

- Amount of variation in the data (variance).
- What error probability can be tolerated.
- Probability, α, of type I error (detection of effect when one does not exist).
- Power, $1 - \beta$, or equivalently the probability of type II error, β (failure to detect an effect when one does exist).
- The magnitude of effect it is desired to detect. The subtler the effect being detected, the larger the sample size needed.

- Precision of estimate of the given effect.
- Sample size is smaller in one-tailed tests than in corresponding two-tailed tests.

Formulae for sample size calculation may involve either:

- Power calculations: The sample is chosen to identify a given difference with specified power and significance. The power is usually set at between 80–95 %. The significance (range 0–1) is the probability of obtaining the observed difference in the absence of a true population difference.
- Precision estimates: The sample is chosen to ensure that the confidence interval obtained is of a specified width.

Box 21 Calculation of power efficiency

Power efficiency = $Np/Nd \times 100$

where Np = the sample size required to obtain the specified power for a specified criterion of significance with a specified difference in means, using a parametric test, and Nd = the sample size to obtain the equivalent effect with a non-parametric test.

Non-parametric tests

Tests of differences between groups (independent samples)

Two samples
1. Categorical data
   - (i) Fisher's exact test
   - (ii) Chi-square test.
2. Numerical data
   - (i) Mann–Whitney U test: two independent samples
   - (ii) Wilcoxon rank sum test: paired samples
   - (iii) Kolmogorov–Smirnov two-sample test
   - (iv) Wald–Wolfowitz runs test.

Multiple groups
   - (i) Kruskal–Wallis analysis of ranks
   - (ii) Median test.

Tests of differences between variables (dependent samples)

Two variables measured in the same or matched sample
   - (i) Sign test
   - (ii) Wilcoxon's matched pairs signed rank test: numerical data
   - (iii) McNemar's test (dichotomous variables): categorical data.

More than two variables measured in the same or matched sample (repeated measures)

   (i)   Friedman's two-way analysis of variance: numerical data

   (ii)   Cochran's Q test: categorical data.

Tests of relationships between variables

1. Categorical data (both):
      (i)   Cramer's contingency coefficient or V
      (ii)   Lambda.
2. Categorical data (one or both):
      (i)   Risk ratio or odds ratio
      (ii)   Logistic regression
      (iii) Chi square
      (iv) Phi coefficient
      (v)   Fisher exact test.
3. Categorical data (three or more sets of variables):
      (i)   Kendall coefficient of concordance: assesses the degree of agreement among m sets of n ranks.
4. Ordinal data (one or both):
      (i)   Spearman rho (rank correlation coefficient)
      (ii)   Kendall tau
      (iii) Gamma statistic
      (iv) Phi coefficient.

Parametric tests

Differences between two or more independent groups

Two groups

1. Normal distribution; Z statistic: population variance known.
2. t test with n – 1 degrees of freedom: population variance unknown.

Three or more groups

1. ANOVA.

Differences between two or more paired (dependent or matched) groups

Two groups

1. Paired t test.

Three or more groups

1. Repeated measures ANOVA.

Association between two variables
1. Numerical (interval or ratio) data (both):
    (i)   Regression (for prediction)
    (ii)   Pearson correlation coefficient (for association).

Tests of agreement between two measurement techniques
1. Categorical data:
    (i)   Kappa statistic.
2. Numerical data:
    (i)   Bland–Altman plot or intraclass coefficient: a bias plot that plots the
           difference between the tests against an estimation of the true result of the
           test (assumed to be the mean of the test results). The mean, mean + 2
           standard deviations, and mean – 2 standard deviations are plotted as
           horizontal line.

Goodness-of-fit tests
These are tests that compare fitted responses obtained from a postulated model
with the observed data.
    The fit is good in the presence of a good agreement between fitted and observed
data. Goodness-of-fit for categorical data is usually measured by the chi-square test
or a likelihood-ratio test.

Statistical hypothesis testing (Neyman–Pearson paradigm)
A statistical hypothesis is a statement about one or more parameters of a population
distribution. It is never a statement about the sample alone.

Steps in hypothesis testing
- State the research hypothesis (a testable belief or opinion).
- State the statistical hypotheses, determining whether a one- or two-tailed test is
  required (i.e. whether it is intended to study differences in one or both
  directions). A one-tailed test halves the probability of a chance result when
  compared to a two-tailed test, i.e. a smaller treatment effect is needed to achieve
  the same level of statistical significance when the treatment effect is in a
  specified direction. A one-tailed test has more power and a lower type II error.
      A two-tailed test is, however, preferable where the direction of the anticipated
  results cannot be predicted, e.g. when the treatment under study can cause either
  benefit or harm.
- State the null hypothesis, which expresses the idea that an observed difference is
  due to chance only. It is a statement that a parameter in a statistical model takes
  a particular value. The working hypothesis is thus one of no difference caused by
  the intervention.
- State the alternative (target) hypothesis, which expresses the manner of deviation
  of the value of a parameter in a statistical model from that specified in the null
  hypothesis.
- Specify the decision rule to evaluate the null hypothesis.

- Specify the test statistic (a measure of difference between the data and what is expected from the null hypothesis),which is analogous to the parameter specified by the null hypothesis. It is a function of the sample data on which the decision to reject or not reject the null hypothesis is based. The sampling distribution for the test statistic is known when the tested hypothesis is true.
- Identify the relevant sampling distribution, and distribution of the test statistic.
- Identify the level of significance (α).
- Determine the critical region of sampling distribution or distribution of test statistic for the given significance level. The size of the rejection region is expressed by the level of significance, α. The location of the rejection region is determined by whether a one-tailed or two-tailed test is used.
- Analyse the data.
- Evaluate the statistics.
- Interpret the statistics.
- Compare the actual value of the test statistic against its critical value.
- Reject the null hypothesis if the test statistic falls in the critical region (region of rejection). This region contains data relatively probable if the null hypothesis is not true.

  For a two-tailed test the test statistic is selected so that the largest and smallest values of the test statistic combined correspond to the rejection region.

  For a one-tailed test, the test statistic is selected so that either and only the largest or smallest values of the test statistic correspond to the rejection region. A one-tailed test should only be used if there is prior knowledge indicating that the relationship being sought can take only one direction.
- If the value of the test statistic falls outside the critical region, the null hypothesis cannot be rejected at the chosen level of significance. The null distribution of the test statistic is the probability distribution when the null hypothesis is assumed to be true.

Box 22 Decision on null hypothesis

Reality	Accept	Reject
True	Correct decision Probability: $1 - \alpha$	Type I error Probability: α (significance level)
False	Type II error Probability: β	Correct decision Probability: $1 - \beta$

The general form of the test statistic is:

$$\frac{\text{Observed statistic} - \text{expected statistic}}{\text{Standard error statistic}}$$

Hypothesis testing may involve means or proportions.

The best test for a simple hypothesis is a test in the set of tests with agreed type I error size (α) that minimises the size of the type II error (β). This depends on the use of a theorem called the **Neyman–Pearson lemma**. The lemma states that the likelihood-ratio test is optimal.

Characteristics of the null hypothesis

- It is either true or not true.
- It cannot be proved, only disproved. It is formulated only for the express purpose of being rejected.
- It anticipates failure.

Calculation of the p value for a statistical test

- The value of the test statistic is determined.
- If a one-tailed test is used, the p value is equal to the tail area beyond the observed value of the test statistic in the same direction as the alternative hypothesis.
- If a two-tailed test is used, the p value is equal to twice the tail area beyond the observed value of the test statistic in the direction of its sign.

Power

Features

- It is a function of the significance level (size of α) adopted.
- It equals $1 - \beta$.
- It represents the probability of correctly rejecting the null hypothesis, i.e. of not making a type II error.
- It equates to the ability to find a difference in distributions when there really is one.
- A test based upon a larger sample size is more powerful.
- A one-tailed test is more powerful than a two-tailed test.
- The power of a test depends on the type of statistical test chosen, sample size, size of experimental effects and the level of error in experimental measurements.

Steps in power analysis

- Specify the form and magnitude of intervention effect worth detecting, based on a judgement on what is clinically significant. The effect size is the size of the difference between the hypothesised means, i.e. between the null hypothesis and the alternative hypothesis.
- Select a test statistic for that effect.
- Determine the distribution of that test statistic under the null hypothesis.
- Select the critical values in that distribution that determine whether or not the investigator will reject the null hypothesis.
- Develop an expression for the variance of the intervention effect under the null hypothesis in terms of parameters that are easily estimated.
- Gather estimates of those parameters.
- Include a sensitivity analysis that varies the estimates of the most important parameters.

The lowest adequate power in respect of a given effect size is defined at 80% (β < 0.2). With 80% power there is an 80% chance of the correct identification of a given effect size being statistically significant.

A small study can demonstrate a statistically significant result if the magnitude of difference between groups is large.

Power curves are used to depict an increase in power with an increase in the value of the difference to be detected and in the sample size.

There is a power function associated with any given sample size that describes the level of power $1 - \beta$ with which any specified difference can be detected.

Multiple testing

This is used in the following circumstances:

- When there are multiple endpoints or outcomes influenced by the same set of explanatory variables.
- Multiple pairwise comparisons, as in ANOVA or multiple regression techniques.
- Secondary analyses.
- Subgroup analyses.

Bonferroni correction

- Guards against an increase in type I error when performing multiple significance tests.
- When testing n independent hypotheses, to maintain the type I error at some selected value α, each of the n tests to be performed is judged against a significance level, α/n. The traditional probability level is divided by the number of dependent variables.
- It is not recommended if more than five tests are to be applied.
- It is conservative as it assumes that the different endpoints are not correlated. This may lead to failure to reject the null hypothesis and to wide confidence intervals.

Other tests for making multiple inferences on the same data: multimean comparison tests or post hoc tests

- Scheffe's test for any and all mean or sum comparisons. It is the most conservative multiple comparison test, requiring a higher critical value to determine significance.
- Duncan multiple-range procedures: ordered comparisons of means arranged in a hierarchy. Significance is based on the number of ordered steps between means.
- Newman–Keuls procedure: The testing of ranked means or sums of experimental intervals tested for significance, based on the number of ordered steps involved in the comparisons. The critical value corresponds to the number of steps between the means. This can only be used for pairwise comparisons.
- Multiple t tests within one set of data increases the likelihood of committing type I error. The Fisher's least significant difference test or protected t test may be used. This test compares each population mean with each other using the t test when the population means are shown to be significantly different with ANOVA.

- Tukey's honestly significant difference method, based on the studentised range statistic. It is only applicable for pairwise comparisons. The studentised range distribution is used for testing all differences among pairs of means, taking into account the number of means under consideration. The larger the number of means under consideration, the larger the critical value.
- Dunnett's procedure: This is used for comparing several treatment means with a single control mean.
- Orthogonal test for comparison between independent sets of means.

t test

Types of t tests
- One-sample *t* test. Tests if the sample mean for a variable differs significantly from the given population with a known mean and unknown variance.
- Unpaired or independent *t* test. Tests if the population means estimated by two independent samples differ significantly
- Paired or related *t* test. Tests if the population means estimated by two dependent samples differ significantly. The subjects are used as their own control groups, as in before and after data, being tested on the same variable. The test is also employed if the two groups are matched on one or more characteristics.

Requirements
The *t* test can be used if:

- The observations are independent.
- The observations are randomly drawn from normally distributed populations.
- These normal populations have the same (homogeneous) variance, or a known ratio of variances.
- The variables are measured in at least an interval scale.

The *t* distribution is leptokurtic, with a greater concentration of values around the mean and in the tails than the normal distribution.

General principles
- The sample means are calculated.
- An estimate of standard deviations of the two parent populations is calculated using the numbers of readings in the two sets of data.
- The value of standard deviation thus obtained is used to estimate the standard error of the differences between the means.
- The value of $m1 - m2$ is divided by the standard error of the means.
- This is looked up in a *t* table to find the probability of obtaining a difference in means $m1 - m2$ as large or larger than this, noting the degrees of freedom.

The magnitude of *t* depends on:

- The observed difference between the means.
- The size of the sample.
- The magnitude of sample variance.

- The significance level or α.
- Whether the test is one-tailed or two-tailed.

t test for independent samples

Method
- Formulate the null hypothesis and alternative hypothesis.
- Check for normal distribution and equality of variance.
- Calculate sample means and the difference between them.
- Calculate pooled best estimate of standard deviation.
- Calculate the standard error of means and the standard error of difference between means.
- Calculate t = difference between sample means/pooled standard error.

t test for paired samples
It is used to determine whether there is a significant difference between the mean values of the same measurement made under two different conditions.

Method
- Formulate the null hypothesis and alternative hypothesis.
- Check for normal distribution and equality of variance.
- Calculate sample means and the difference between them.
- Calculate best estimate of standard deviation of differences between paired variables.
- Calculate standard error of mean difference between samples.
- Calculate t = difference between means/standard error of differences.
- Calculate number of degrees of freedom.
- Choose level of significance and hence critical value of t.
- If t is greater than the critical value, reject the null hypothesis.

Degrees of freedom

Characteristics
- The size reflects the number of observations that are free to vary after certain restrictions have been placed on the data, still leaving the sole sample with certain relevant characteristics. These restrictions are inherent in the organisation of the data.
- The degrees of freedom for any statistic is equal to the number of independent quantities used in calculation of the statistic (sample size) minus the number of parameters in the statistic estimated from them.
- The degrees of freedom for a variance are 1 less than the sample size. They quantify the amount of information available in a data set for estimation of the population variance.
- Any statistic that does not make a correction for loss of independence, or freedom, is a biased estimate of its population parameter. This is because the laws of chance assume the independence of observations, i.e. they assume freedom to vary.

Calculations
- For goodness-of-fit tests with n classes, $df = n - 1$.
- For goodness-of-fit tests to a binomial or Poisson distribution with n classes, $df = n - 2$.
- For goodness-of-fit tests to a normal distribution with n classes, $df = n - 3$.
- For tests of association for a contingency table with m rows and n columns, $df = (n - 1), (m - 1)$.

Chi-square test

Karl Pearson introduced the chi-square test in 1900 and applied it to test goodness-of-fit for frequencies. He derived chi-square in terms of a correlated multivariate normal distribution. He extended its uses to testing for independence in contingency tables in 1904.

The chi-square test may be regarded as both:

- A test of goodness-of-fit, i.e. how well the observed frequency distribution fits a hypothetical expected frequency distribution. It is used for multinomial populations, where each member of the population is assigned to one, and only one, of several classes or categories. The test ascertains whether a significant difference exists between an observed number of objects or responses falling in each category and an expected number based upon the null hypothesis. The closer the expected number is to the observed number across all cells, the less likelihood is there of the difference being statistically significant. By squaring the differences the direction of the difference is ignored.
- A test of association or of independence, i.e. for existence or non-existence of a relationship between nominal or categorical variables (in the form of counts).

Requirements
- The data must be in the form of frequencies counted in each of a number of categories (percentages or proportions cannot be used) which are mutually exclusive – i.e. univariate categorical data.
- The total numbers observed must exceed 20.
- The expected frequency under the null hypothesis in any one category or cell must be more than 5.
- The data should represent a random sample of independent observations from a multinomial population.
- The observed frequencies differ from the expected frequencies with more than two possible outcomes.
- No ranking of data is required.
- No assumptions are made regarding normal distribution of the data. The deviations (observed – expected values) are expected to demonstrate a normal distribution.
- The groups compared must be of approximately the same size.

Contingency table
- A table of counts showing the frequencies with which two random variables presented simultaneously take various values in a sample.
- It is used to summarise the relationship between two categorical variables.
- A table is constructed in which each item is classified twice – in columns and in rows. All levels of one variable are listed as rows, and all levels of the other variable as columns.
- The sum of all cell frequencies is equal to the number of subjects used.
- Both rows and columns totals are calculated: these are the marginal totals.
- Estimates of cell means (expected frequencies) are calculated:

$$\frac{\text{Row total} \times \text{column total}}{\text{Total number of observations}}$$

- The differences between expected and observed cell frequencies for each cell are squared.
- Chi-square is computed, using the formula:

$$\chi^2 = \Sigma_{\text{all cells}} \frac{(O - E)^2}{E}$$

where O = observed count, E = expected count.
- The degrees of freedom $(r - 1)(c - 1)$ are determined, where r = number of rows, c = number of columns. This is the only parameter needed to specify any chi-square distribution.
- In the absence of a relationship between column and row totals, the observed frequencies differ from the expected frequencies by a small amount, and the computed chi-square statistic assumes a small value.
- The presence of a relationship between column and row totals leads to substantial variation between observed and expected frequencies, leading to a large value for the computed chi-square statistic.

Yates' continuity correction for a 2×2 contingency table
- Subtract 0.5 from the absolute value of the difference between observed and expected frequency before squaring.
- Adjust the other cells so that row and column totals remain constant. This leads to a reduction in the size of chi-square.
- This reduces discrepancy between the calculated chi-square statistic and theoretical chi-square attribution. A calculated chi-square is based on frequencies (which are whole numbers) and varies in discrete jumps. The chi-square table, representing the distributions of chi-square, gives values from a continuous scale.

In general, the correction is only made when the number of degrees of freedom is $v = 1$. The need for this correction is however felt to be uncertain and is probably only indicated in the presence of fixed marginal (row and column) totals. Use of the correction may lead to the failure of rejection of a false null hypothesis.

Fisher exact probability test for 2 × 2 tables

Requirements
- Discrete data (nominal or ordinal).
- Two independent samples, small in size.
- The scores are obtained from two independent random samples.
- All fall into one or other of two mutually exclusive classes (take only two possible values), i.e. dichotomous data.
- Every subject in both groups obtains one of two possible scores.

Method
- The scores are represented by frequencies in a 2 × 2 contingency table. At least one of the expected cell frequencies is less than 5. The row and column totals (marginal totals) are assumed to be the same on the observed data.
- The null hypothesis of independence between row and column variables is that the observed frequencies could occur by chance. It is rejected at the 5% level of significance if the calculated value of the probability is less than 0.05.
- The exact probability, without use of an approximation, of getting any particular values of the variables is given by a hypergeometric formula. The assumption is that the conditional distribution of the value in the upper left hand cell of the table is a hypergeometric distribution.
- The test evaluates the probabilities associated with all possible 2 × 2 tables with the same row and column (marginal) totals as the observed data.

Box 23 Display of data in Fisher exact 2 × 2 probability tables

	Positive	Negative	Total
Group I	A	B	A + B
Group II	C	D	C + D
Totals	A + C	B + D	A + B + C + D = N

P is equal to the sum of the factorial calculation repeated for each possible arrangement of the values in the cells showing an association equal to or stronger than that between the two variables.

$$P = \frac{(A+B)!(C+D)!(A+C)!(B+D)!}{N!\,A!\,B!\,CD!}$$

The factorial of a number is the product of that number multiplied by a series of numbers, each being 1 smaller than the preceding number.

Cochran's *Q* test for related observations

Use
- To detect if there is a significant difference between three or more sets of matched observations, when the responses are dichotomous (e.g. present/absent, cured/nor cured).
- The chi-square test is not applicable as the samples are not independent.

Method
- r items are tested in c ways. Each of c treatments is applied independently to each of r subjects or blocks.
- Positive responses are recorded as 1, and negative responses as 0.
- The data is arranged in a table with r rows and c columns of 1's and 0's.
- The hypothesis is that the probabilities of positive responses for the columns are equal.
- If the hypothesis is true and r is large, the statistic Q has approximately a chi-square distribution with $c - 1$ degrees of freedom.
- At the level of significance the hypothesis will be rejected if $Q > x1 - \alpha(c - 1)^2$.

Assumptions
- The subjects are randomly selected from the population of all possible subjects.
- Treatment responses may be dichotomised in a manner common to all treatments in each subject or block.

Odds ratio
This can be used as an estimation technique for categorical data, especially in 2×2 contingency tables. Confidence intervals may be constructed around the odds ratio.

Measurement of agreement of categorical data: kappa
Kappa is a measure of interobserver agreement that is beyond the agreement expected based on chance alone, i.e. a chance-corrected measure of agreement. It is the ratio of the agreement actually observed minus the agreement expected by chance, divided by 1 (which corresponds to perfect agreement) minus the agreement expected by chance.

The kappa statistic runs from -1 to $+1$. If the agreement is totally by chance, the expected value is zero. It is equal to $+1$ if there is complete agreement between the two categories. A value of -1 indicates total disagreement.

Kappa can be calculated from the observed and expected frequencies in the diagonal of a 2×2 or a square $r \times c$ contingency table (in which the numbers of r's and c's are the same).

A weighted kappa assigns weights to the observed agreement and the chance observed agreement. It is usually higher than the unweighted kappa. This is most

---

Box 24 Calculation of kappa

$$\kappa = \frac{Pa - Pc}{1 - Pc}$$

Pa = observed proportion of agreement or concordant diagnoses
Pc = proportion of agreement or concordant diagnoses expected on the basis of chance.

Box 25 Strength of agreement of kappa values

κ values	Strength of agreement
> 0.20	Poor
0.21–0.40	Fair
0.41–0.60	Moderate
0.61–0.80	Good
0.81–1.00	Very good

suitable for ordered categories but there is controversy as to whether it should be used at all.

Kappa can be extended to use for more than one rater comparison, and for polychotomous rather than dichotomous variables.

Kappa is not a measure of validity.

Sign test

This test is used to test one-sided hypotheses concerning medians relating to small samples drawn from non-normally distributed populations.

Requirements

- Independent pairs of observations in two things being compared (e.g. treatments).
- Each of the two observations of a given pair has been made under similar conditions.
- The different pairs have been observed in different conditions.
- Ideally, no ties occur in paired comparisons. If they do, they should be excluded, with a consequent reduction in sample size.

Method

- X and Y represent measurements made on A and B.
- The number of pairs of observations is N.
- N pairs of observations and their differences are denoted by $(X1,Y1),(X2,Y2), \ldots$ (XN,YN) and $X1 - Y1, X2 - Y2, \ldots XN - YN$.
- The test is based on the signs of these differences, di, i.e. the test statistic is the number of positive (or negative) signs associated with the differences.
- The letter r denotes the number of times the less frequent sign occurs.
- The null hypothesis is that there is the same number of positive and negative signs.
- The test disregards the size or magnitude of the differences, but examines whether the direction of the difference is sufficiently consistent to indicate a real change over time.
- The number of positive differences has a binomial distribution with parameters n and p.

Mann–Whitney U test

A non-parametric test to decide whether two independent samples come from identical populations or whether these populations have unequal distributions, in terms of shape and location (unrelated design).

Requirements

- The samples must be randomly and independently drawn from the respective populations. They need not contain the same numbers of observations. The variable of interest must be continuous.
- The measurement scale should be at least ordinal.
- The distributions of the two sampled populations should differ, if at all, only with respect to location.

Method
- Formulate the null hypothesis and alternative hypothesis and decide on the rejection level.
- Determine the values of $n1$ (number of cases in the smaller group) and $n2$ (number of cases in the larger group).
- Rank the data jointly in an increasing (or decreasing) order of magnitude as a single series of ranks (as if they were in fact one sample), regardless of their signs. However, the distinction between samples from the two groups is preserved by recording the group membership in an adjacent column. A rank of 1 is assigned to the score, which is algebraically lowest.
- If there are ties among observed values belonging to different samples assign each of the tied observations the mean of the ranks which they jointly occupy.
- The null hypothesis is that both samples come from identical populations, i.e. the means of the ranks assigned to the values of the two samples is similar. The number of times a score from one sample is ranked higher than a score from the other sample is similar. The two samples should appear in random order in the joint ranking.
- The alternative hypothesis is that the populations have unequal means. The larger the difference in means, the more likely it is that the majority of the smaller ranks will go to the values of one sample and the higher ranks will go to the values of the other sample.
- If $n1$ and $n2$ are both greater than 20, the sampling distribution of U can be approximated closely with a normal distribution. The U statistic can then be transformed into t or z scores.
- If computed U exceeds the critical value for U at the specified significance level, the null hypothesis can be rejected in favour of the alternative hypothesis.

> **Box 26** Calculation of the U statistic
>
> $$U = n1n2 + \frac{n1(n1 + 1)}{2} - R1$$
>
> where $n1$ and $n2$ are the sizes of the two samples, $R1$ is the sum of the ranks assigned to values of the first sample
>
> or
>
> $$U = n1n2 + \frac{n2(n2 + 1)}{2} - R2$$
>
> where $R2$ is the sum of ranks assigned to values of the second sample.

Wilcoxon matched-pairs signed-ranks test
A non-parametric test used when the same or matched subjects perform under both experimental conditions (related design). It is applied either to paired ranked data or to paired measured non-normal data, to test the null hypothesis that the paired observations do not differ, i.e. the median difference in paired data is zero.

Requirements
- The samples must be random.
- The variable of interest must be continuous.
- The population must be symmetrically distributed about its mean.

- The measurement scale must be at least interval.
- There should be at least six differences that are not zero before a 5% probability level can be reached.
- The test makes use of both the direction (sign) and the magnitude of differences between observations.

Method
- Formulate the null hypothesis and the alternative hypothesis and decide on the rejection level.
- The subjects in the two samples are pooled and ordered in terms of their scores on an ordinal scale
- The differences between the pairs of scores are calculated and given the appropriate plus or minus sign (the absolute value).
- Pairs that show no difference are dropped from the analysis, and the value of n is reduced accordingly.
- The differences are ranked in order of magnitude from the smallest to the largest without respect to sign.
- Tied differences are assigned the average of the tied ranks.
- The ranks corresponding to the different signs are added together separately.
- The test statistic W is the smaller of the sum of the ranks with the same sign, i.e. the sum of the ranks with the less frequent sign.

Wald–Wolfowitz runs test for two samples

Requirements
- The comparison of two unmatched samples.
- Each observation is paired with a numerical score.
- The scores represent a continuously distributed variable.

Method
- There are $N1$ and $N2$ observations respectively in the two samples.
- All observations are drawn independently and at random.
- Observations from sample 1 are called A's and those from sample 2 are called B's.
- All observations are arranged in order, irrespective of the experimental group they come from, in order of magnitude.
- There will be an pattern of observations from the two samples, including runs or clusters of A's and B's.
- For groups of the same size N there can be no more than $2N$ runs in all when the scores from the groups are ordered.
- If the experimental groups are random samples from identical population distributions there would be many runs. If the populations are different there would be less tendency for runs in the sample ordering.

Limitations
- If there are numerous cross-group tied scores this test should not be used.

McNemar change test or test for correlated proportions

Requirements
- This is applicable to nominal or ordinal binary or dichotomous variables.
- The McNemar test for the significance of changes is applicable to 'before and after' designs in which each subject is used as its own control and in which the measurements are made on either a nominal or ordinal scale. These represent paired samples.
- It is a test of the equality of two proportions in cases where each sample proportion involves some of the same observations, making the two sample proportions dependent.

Method
- A fourfold table (2 × 2 table) of frequencies is used to represent the first and second sets of responses from the same individuals. If the total number of people whose responses changed is less than 10, use the binomial test rather than the McNemar test.
- Concordant pairs give no information on the relationship between a factor and its outcome. The test is not based on the number of agreements.
- The test compares the observed proportion of discordant pairs, i.e. untied pairs, with the one factor present and the other absent among all discordant pairs to 0.5.
- The null hypothesis is that the paired proportions are equal.
- The test statistic follows a chi-square distribution with one degree of freedom. It is described by the formula:

$$X^2 (1) = \frac{[(b - c) - 1]^2}{b + c}$$

where b and c are the frequencies in the cells corresponding to discordant pairs.

Epidemiological concepts

Epidemiology refers to the study of health and disease in populations. This clearly differentiates it from the elements of curative medicine that deal with disease in the individual. The processes of quantification, measurement and comparison of health status warrant a close link with appropriate statistical techniques. The data for epidemiological studies is derived from either routinely collected morbidity and mortality statistics, or from specially designed clinical studies or surveys.

Some of the major elements of epidemiology relate to:

- Measurement of the health status of populations and evaluation of their health care needs.
- The study of patterns of disease in defined population groups.
- The investigation of the natural history (cause, progression and outcome) of disease, to allow insight into prevention.
- Measuring the efficacy of health care interventions.
- Defining priorities for the use of scarce medical resources.
- The identification of high risk groups for disease, including occupational risks.
- Studies of the association between environmental agents or conditions and the development of specific diseases.

Clinical study design
The study can be either:

- Observational or experimental.
- Prospective or retrospective.
- Longitudinal or cross-sectional (concurrent).
- And can involve either single or multiple samples.

Study types

Observational
1. Non-controlled:
     (i)   Case report
     (ii)   Case studies.
2. Controlled:
     (i)   Case-control: retrospective/cross-sectional
     (ii)   Survey: cross-sectional/retrospective
     (iii) Cohort (prospective/longitudinal/retrospective/cross-sectional)
     (iv)   Ecological studies.

Experimental (interventional): longitudinal
1. Randomised.
2. Non-randomised:
     (i)   Literature controls
     (ii)   Historical controls
     (iii) Concurrent controls.

Observational studies

The exposure is not assigned to the individual subject by the investigator.

Case reports and case series
Although regarded as low level evidence, case reports and series have a role in the following situations:

- The recognition and description of new disease.
- The recognition of side effects of treatment, which may be either beneficial or detrimental.
- The recognition of rare manifestations of disease.
- Further characterisation of rare or unusual diseases.
- The recognition of phenomena which lead to hypothesis generation and confirmation by formalised test procedures.
- Case series can provide the case group for case-control studies.

Case-control study
- The cases and controls are matched with respect to confounding variables. The matching criteria can be age, sex, social class, level of physical activity, etc. This increases efficiency and reduces the required sample size, and improves the comparability of the collected data.
- Control of confounding requires stratification by levels of the confounding variable(s) whether or not matching has been achieved.
- The cases have the outcome of interest, while the controls do not.
- Cases and controls are studied to look for any differences in past exposure to

possible causes of the disease (generally retrospective), i.e. one works back from outcome to exposure. There may be recall bias on past exposure amongst cases. The exposure to the risk factor must not be rare.

- These studies do not estimate incidence or prevalence and cannot be used to calculate incidence rates, relative risks or attributable risks.
- Odds ratios are used to measure association with exposure.

The categories that can be defined are:

- Cases:
  Exposed
  Not exposed.
- Controls:
  Exposed
  Not exposed.

Nested case-control study

A case-control study nested within a large defined cohort, from which cases and controls are chosen and for which information on exposures and risk factors are already available.

Some or all of the additional information needed for the analysis is collected only after the outcome of interest has been observed. All cases identified in the cohort become cases for the nested study. Controls are then selected from a random sample of all participants at risk at the time of occurrence of the cases, thus using only a subset of the cohort. These controls have not developed the outcome, and are matched to the cases by age, sex and other categories.

This design eliminates recall bias and is more economical to perform. By reducing the number of study subjects, the costs of expensive measurements for predictor variables is minimised.

Cohort study (follow-up or incidence study)

- Two groups, one exposed and one not exposed to the postulated causative factor, are followed longitudinally. The exposure must be clearly defined, specific and measurable.
- The study may be completely prospective, retrospective (using secondary data) or ambispective (combining existing records with further prospective follow-up).
- Types of cohorts include age, date of birth, marriage, occupational (exposure), disease and intervention (preventive and therapeutic) cohorts.
- The two groups are not randomised.
- There may be attrition of the study population over the follow-up period from migration, lack of participation and death.
- True incidence rates, relative risks and attributable risks can be calculated.

The classical example of a cohort study is the long-term follow-up of male British general practitioners and their smoking habits, which has confirmed the strong association between cigarette smoking and the development of lung cancer.

Cross-sectional study (survey or prevalence study)
- A defined population is studied at a single time interval. Cases and controls come from the same clinical population. Exposure and disease state are measured simultaneously.
- This type of study can be used to determine the prevalence of disease and its characteristics.
- No information is provided about long-term outcomes.

Ecological study
- This involves collection of information about one or more characteristics of a clearly defined population and relating to the number of individuals that form the population.
- The population may be defined according to geographical, geopolitical or time criteria.
- The study design is useful in the generation of hypotheses.

Experimental studies

An experiment is a study in which only the independent variable is manipulated and all other variables are maintained constant. This eliminates all possible factors that might influence the effect being measured other than the one under study.

A standardised procedure is necessary. Subjects are allocated randomly to the different experimental conditions. The effect of the intervention on certain predetermined outcomes is ascertained.

Designs of experimental studies

Related designs
The results in one group are directly related to the results in the other group.

1. Repeated measures (within-subject or treatment-by-subject design): The same group is tested in both experimental conditions, each subject acting as his or her own control. Multiple measurements are thus made on the same experimental subject. An order effect may confound the results, by improvements in subject performance or by boredom or fatigue. An order effect may be minimised by:
   (i) Counterbalancing the experimental conditions between the groups
   (ii) Randomising the stimulus items and mixing them together
   (iii) Giving time between the experimental conditions to minimise carry-over effects from the first intervention.
2. Matched pairs: Two different groups are used to test the experimental conditions. This is necessary when testing differences between two different groups, and when employing control groups. Some subject variables may still be present as it is difficult to find perfect matches.

Unrelated designs

The results in one group are unrelated to the results in the other group.

1. **Single participant:** All the experimental trials are conducted on the same subject. This is useful when few subjects are available.
2. **Independent samples:** A different group is tested in different experimental conditions. This means that:
   (i) Subject variables are not controlled
   (ii) More study subjects may be needed
   (iii) Non-parametric tests may be required owing to lack of homogeneity of variance.

Evidence supporting causality

- Size of effect: relative risk.
- Strength of association: p value (estimate of the probability of rejecting the null hypothesis); odds ratio; relative risk.
- Dose-response: a larger exposure to the cause is associated with a higher disease rate, and a reduction in exposure with a lower disease rate.
- Consistency of association: internal validity; confirmed by repeated observations in studies using different methods.
- Replication of results: external validity.
- Specificity of association: one cause leads to one effect.
- Temporality: proper time sequence, with cause preceding effect.
- Biological gradient.
- Biological plausibility: the association makes sense.
- Coherence of evidence: the association explains other observations about the disease, e.g. age and sex distribution.
- Experimental evidence.
- Analogy: analogous to well-established causative exposure for disease.

Box 27 Causes of apparent associations

Bias
Chance
Confounding

Odds ratio

It is an estimate of the association between an exposure (risk factor) and an outcome (disease), which can be considered as two dichotomous random variables. The number of individuals with a disease is expressed relative to the number without the characteristic. The odds of an event are the number of events divided by the number of non-events.

If the probability of an event is p, then the odds of that event is $o = p/(1 - p)$. It is thus a quotient of two probabilities, i.e. the probability of an event divided by the probability of a non-event.

If a sequence of Bernoulli trials are performed in which an outcome of interest occurs a times and does not occur b times ($n = a + b$), then the odds of the outcome of interest are a/b.

An odds ratio is obtained by dividing the odds in the treated or exposed group by the odds in the control group. With a dichotomous exposure, a 2×2 table can be drawn up and the odds ratio calculated as the ratio of the 'cross-products'.

Odds ratio is used in epidemiological studies to describe the likely harm an exposure might cause, producing an odds ratio greater than 1. Odds ratios are ideal to give an estimate of risk for case-control studies, where disease prevalence is not known.

In clinical trials of new treatments which reduce event rates, an odds ratio of less than one is sought.

For rare events, odds ratios and relative risks are similar. The odds ratio overestimates the magnitude of both harmful associations (relative risk > 1) and protective associations (relative risk < 1). As the outcome becomes more frequent, the odds ratio and the relative risk diverge. The comparison of risk represented by the odds ratio does not depend on whether the investigator chooses to determine the risk of an event occurring or not occurring. Odds ratios can be combined across strata using Mantel–Haenszel methods.

> **Box 28** Calculation of the odds ratio from a case-control study using a 2×2 table
>
> | | Disease + | Disease − |
> |---|---|---|
> | Exposure + | a | b |
> | Exposure − | c | d |
>
> Odds of exposure among those with disease = a/c
> Odds of exposure among the controls = b/d
> OR = $(a/c)/(b/d)$
>   = $a/c \times d/b$ (cross-products ratio)

Log transformation of the odds ratio

The odds ratio is a multiplicative measure of association, and has an asymmetrical distribution.

The logarithmic transformation of the odds ratio yields a nearly symmetrical distribution, which is approximated by a normal distribution. The log-odds is an additive measure of association. A log-odds ratio of 0 implies absence of association. Positive and negative values reflect corresponding degrees of association.

Berkson's fallacy

The use of non-random samples will lead to odds ratios that demonstrate a non-existent relationship among variables. This can occur with case-control studies in which there are differential rates of hospital admission for cases and controls.

Neyman's bias

An incidence or prevalence bias that arises when a gap in time is interposed between exposure and selection of study participants. An unrepresentative case group may be created when studying diseases that are transient, rapidly fatal or subclinical.

Relative risk

The ratio of:

$$\frac{\text{Incidence of disease in the exposed group}}{\text{Incidence of disease in the non-exposed (control) group}}$$

Alternative, the ratio of:

$$\frac{\text{Probability of the outcome if the risk factor is present}}{\text{Probability of the outcome if the risk factor is absent}}$$

The relative risk approaches the odds ratio as the disease becomes increasingly rare.

Box 29 Calculation of the relative risk from a cohort study using a 2 × 2 table

	Disease +	Disease −
Exposure +	a	b
Exposure −	c	d

Risk of disease with exposure to risk factor= $a/(a + b)$
Risk of disease without exposure to risk factor= $c/(c + d)$

$RR = a/(a + b)/c(c + d)$

$RR = 1$ no association between disease and exposure
$RR > 1$ greater risk in exposed group of disease; exposure may be causal
$RR < 1$ lesser risk in exposed group of disease; exposure may be protective

---

Absolute risk reduction

The difference in the risk of an event between experimental and control groups.

Number needed to treat

The number of patients who must be treated to prevent one patient from experiencing the adverse effects of the disease being studied (e.g. death, stroke). It is the inverse of the attributable benefit, i.e. the number of events prevented for each number treated.

Does not provide a population perspective, i.e. state that the total population will benefit from applying the intervention. The lower the number needed to treat, the better the treatment.

Likelihood ratio

The proportion of patients with the disease with a positive test divided by the proportion of patients without the disease with a positive test gives the positive likelihood ratio. The larger this is, the better the test is at diagnosing the target disorder.

The proportion of patients with the disease with a negative test divided by the proportion of patients without the disease with a negative test gives the negative likelihood ratio. The smaller this is, the better the test is at excluding the target disorder.

The likelihood ratio allows usage of all information in a test and can be used to describe the performance of a diagnostic test.

For dichotomous tests the likelihood ratio for a positive test is sensitivity/(1 – specificity) and the likelihood ratio for a negative test is (1 – sensitivity/specificity).

Crossover trial

Each patient receives two or more treatments in sequence, where one of the treatments may be a placebo or no treatment. Each patient thus acts as his or her own control. The trial should have a randomised design, with assignment to a given order of treatment and control at random.

The design is applicable to chronic conditions with no lasting cure. The condition being studied should be reasonably stable over time. The treatment should not have a long-term effect, as with surgical interventions.

Problems may arise with:

- Carryover therapeutic effects (pharmacological or psychological) of the first treatment.
- Period effects as the disease may progress, regress or fluctuate in severity during the investigation period.

Two types of previously specified crossover rules may be used – either involving a change in treatments after a specified length of time (time dependent) or involving a crossover when indicated by the clinical characteristics of the patient (disease-state dependent).

An extension of the crossover design is the **n-of-1 trial**, where each patient is given multiple courses of the study treatments in a random sequence, with appropriate washout periods between treatments. The study outcome is assessed at the end of each treatment period. This allows determining consistency of response to a particular treatment.

An **enriched enrollment design** is useful for the study of treatments to which only a small proportion of patients respond. Responders are entered into a series of comparisons between treatment and placebo.

Randomised controlled trial (RCT) design

- Determine eligibility for entry to the study.
- Obtain informed consent.
- Randomise after consent is obtained.
- Exclude subjects who do not consent.
- Randomly allocate subjects to receive either the new treatment or the standard treatment or placebo (the latter two groups comprise the control group).

Box 29A

Study population → Random sample → Sample population → Random allocation → Experimental/control group

Pragmatic randomised controlled trials are often preferrable as they reflect the homogeneity of the study population by minimising exclusion criteria and by defining patient groups by presentation rather than by final diagnosis.

Evaluation of randomised trial design

Background information for trial
- Motivation, i.e. the need to perform the trial.
- Funding sources; any consequent conflict of interests.
- Review of relevant literature.
- Pilot study.

Design
- Objectives: specific hypotheses stated.
- Diagnostic criteria for entry to the trial (inclusion and exclusion criteria).
- Informed consent during enrolment of subjects.
- Use of concurrent control subjects.
- Use of well-defined treatments or interventions.
- Random allocation to treatment: removes potential bias in allocation to intervention or to control group, and covariates balance between the intervention and control groups.
- Method of randomisation described: e.g. random number generator, computer, random number tables, shuffled cards, tossed coins. Inadequate methods include alternate assignment, assignment by odd or even birth date, by day of the week, by date of admission or by hospital number. The investigator will often not be blinded to the intervention with these methods resulting in bias. Central computerised telephone, fax or email randomisation is currently the best method available for determining treatment allocation. Other methods of random allocation include the use of sequentially numbered, sealed and opaque envelopes, and sequentially numbered containers.
- Incorporation of blindness to treatment when appropriate: reduces measurement bias in the assessor and bias due to the placebo effect in the subject.
- Criteria for outcome measures. It may be cheaper and easier in some situations to use surrogate markers in place of the endpoint of primary interest.
- Power-based assessment of the adequacy of sample size.
- Duration of post-treatment follow-up.
- Comparability of treatment and control groups.
- Completeness of follow-up. All drop-outs accounted for. All subjects accounted for and attributed at conclusion of trial.
- Side effects of treatment accounted for.

Trial analysis
- Appropriate statistical analyses.
- Confidence intervals given for the main results.
- All clinically important outcomes reported.
- Size and precision of treatment effect described. The precision of estimate of

treatment effect size depends on the number of randomised subjects and on the size of the treatment effect.

- Intention to treat analysis: subjects are analysed in the group they were originally randomly allocated to, not in the way they were actually treated. This accounts for those who leave the study early, take other excluded medications or are non-compliant. This avoids the distortion of the balance of extraneous variables that is achieved by randomisation. The bias introduced by compliance may relate to outcome. An efficacy analysis in which only subjects who complied with the randomised treatment are studied may be associated with bias in favour of the treatment. However, intention to treat analysis may also lead to underestimation of the true treatment effect, caused by inclusion of non-compliers.

  Lack of compliance with treatment may be related to discomfort or side effects associated with treatment, the level of effort required by the patient, as well as perceptions of the value of the treatment.
- Justifiable conclusions.
- Applicability of study findings.

Randomised consent design
- This design reduces the risk of low rates of subject consent especially associated with experimental study designs involving new forms of invasive treatment.
- Randomisation occurs initially.
- Informed consent is obtained only from the group allocated to receive the experimental treatment.
- This group is further divided into those subjects who accept the experimental treatment, and those who refuse consent to this treatment and thereby receive the standard treatment.
- There are, however, ethical problems associated with a study design in which not all subjects receive informed consent.

Problems associated with randomised controlled trials
- Cost.
- The need for large sample sizes.
- Ethical issues, e.g. informed consent.

A randomised clinical trial may be unethical if:
- Informed consent is not obtained.
- A placebo is used when standard therapy is effective.
- If significant risks are imposed on subjects without a realistic estimate of substantial benefit.

Confounding factors
Factors other than the intervention under study that can affect the evolution of a patient's condition following the administration of therapy:

- Regression to the mean, where the improvement is a purely statistical phenomenon, i.e. even if the treatment is ineffective.

- Spontaneous worsening or improvement of the disease.
- The effects of concomitant therapies.
- The placebo effect.

Confounding can hide a real effect or lead to a spurious treatment effect. **Simpson's paradox** refers to reversal of the association between exposure and outcome produced by a confounding factor. This is caused by failure to control for the confounder effect. The effects of two variables (explanatory or extraneous) on a response variable are said to be confounded when they cannot be distinguished from one another. A confounding variable must be associated with the risk factor and causally related to the outcome.

Confounding can be confirmed by stratified analysis, which assesses the effect of a variable on the outcome while keeping another variable constant. In the presence of confounding, there will be a statistically significant difference in the odds ratios derived from the unstratified analysis, which will not be replicated in the stratified analysis.

A propensity score is a weighted combination of potential confounders.

Methods of controlling confounding

In study design
- Restriction in terms of age, race, sex, geographical location, etc., i.e. using exclusion and inclusion criteria.
- Matching for major confounders: pairwise matching of cases and controls.
- Randomisation to control for known and unknown confounders.

In study analysis
- Restriction.
- Stratification: forming strata of data based on the suspected confounding factor. This can be done after completion of the study.
- Multivariate methods to adjust for confounding.
- Demonstration of comparability of confounders between study groups.

Hawthorne effect
- The process of some clinical trials may result in more favourable outcomes in participants irrespective of the type of treatment being tested. This effect was first noted with improvements in the productivity of workers subjected to varying physical conditions, at the Hawthorne works of the Western Electric Company in Chicago during 1924–27.
- The effect can be minimised by randomisation of allocation and by inclusion of a suitable control group.

Placebos

A placebo is a sham or inert treatment. It should be indistinguishable from the pharmacologically active treatment in physical appearance (size, shape, weight, texture), colour, smell and taste.

The effects of placebo can be categorised as follows:

- Meta-analysis suggests that there is no significant effect of placebo as compared with no treatment in pooled data from trials with subjective or objective binary or continuous objective outcomes.
- A significant difference between placebo and no treatment is demonstrable in trials with continuous subjective outcomes and in trials involving the treatment of pain.

Placebos must not be administered when there is a currently available standard and effective treatment. An active placebo is a placebo with properties that simulate the side effects of the active treatment.

Types of blinding
- Unblinded (open label).
- Single blind: only the investigator is aware of the intervention.
- Double blind: neither subjects nor investigators know the identity of the assignment of the intervention.
- Triple blind: the committee monitoring the response variables is unaware of the identity of the groups derived from a double blind trial.

Problems of double-blind trials
- Matching of drugs or other interventions.
- Visual discrepancies in size, shape, colour, texture.
- Differences in odour.
- Differences in taste.
- Differences in weight or specific gravity of tablets.
- Labelling of individual drug bottles or vials.
- Unblinding caused by side effects, accident or by laboratory errors.
- Assessment of blindness, from guesses by subjects.

Limitations of historical controls

Treatment and control groups may not be comparable:
- Criteria for patient selection are not well defined, with the patient groups under comparison not being precisely similar.
- Changes in the natural history of the disease.
- Changes in pathological definitions or staging procedures for the disease.
- Changes in referral patterns.
- The investigator may be more selective than the past physicians in selection of patients for the new treatment.

Experimental environment may not be comparable:
- Inferior quality and incompleteness of recorded data for historical controls.
- Criteria for response may differ between the two patient groups, and may be difficult to ascertain consistently in the historical control group.
- Close monitoring and improved ancillary patient care may improve the new treatment.

The use of historical controls is thus likely to accentuate the effects of a new treatment.

Subgroup analysis

Baseline data are collected on each subject who enters a randomised trial at the time of randomisation. These data relate to demographic features, medical history, ongoing symptoms, physical findings and quantitative diagnostic measures. Subgroup analysis refers to reanalysis of the data on treatment differences using subsamples of patients defined according to subcategories of one or more baseline variables. The categorisation can be decided on before (a priori), preferably, or after (post hoc) the trial has been completed. A priori subgroups must be identifiable from baseline characteristics. Post hoc subgroups can only be used for hypothesis generation.

The problems with subgroup analysis include:

- Low power for detecting an interaction.
- The risk of spurious findings (data dredging) from multiple statistical inferences.
- The risk of unbalanced subgroups, with lack of similarity of the treated and control patients in the subgroups.
- Lack of validity, owing to fewer patients and wider confidence intervals.

If a group of n subjects is divided at random into k equal-sized groups, then the difference between the largest and the smallest subgroup means has an expected value that is approximately k times the standard error of the mean of the whole group (when k is not more than 15).

Problems arise particularly when the trial data are stratified according to several different characteristics recorded after randomisation, without any clear a priori hypothesis, i.e. with post hoc subgroup analyses.

Appropriateness of statistical analysis

- Does the hypothesis predict difference or correlation?
- What is the type of data?
- If continuous data, is it normally distributed?
- If categorical data, is it summarised as a proportion or a percentage?
- Is the design related or unrelated?

Errors in analysis

- Lack of a clearly defined hypothesis.
- Inappropriate study design.
- Misclassification of data.
- Improper assumptions of independence among the data.
- Failure to report specific statistical tests.
- Failure to report exact P values associated with the chosen test.
- Failure to report confidence intervals.

Cluster (group) randomisation trial

A trial in which clusters, or intact social units, are randomised to different intervention groups. Participants are asked for consent to treatment, but not to randomisation.

A loss of statistical efficiency occurs compared with trials that randomise individuals to intervention groups. This is because the responses of individuals in an intact cluster are more similar than the responses of individuals in different clusters.

An intraclass or interclass correlation coefficient is needed for study subjects within clusters as an estimate of the effect of clustering. An intraclass correlation coefficient is the proportion of between-person variance relative to the total variance from two sources: between-person variance and within-person variance (differences between measurements within individuals who are sampled).

The design may be used to reduce the risk of contamination bias associated with individual randomisation. Contamination of control participants reduces the point estimate of an intervention's effectiveness. This may lead to a type II error.

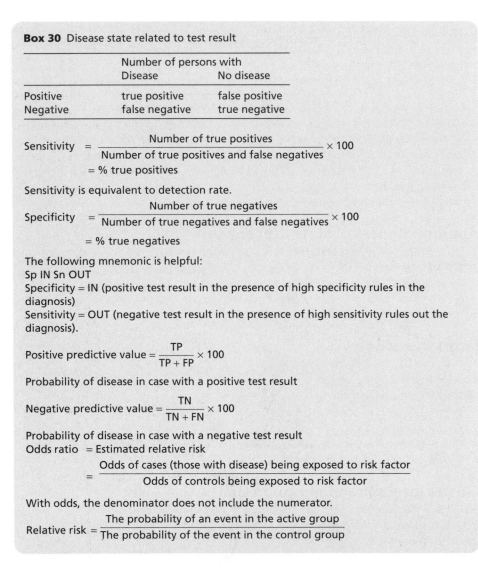

Box 30 Disease state related to test result

	Number of persons with	
	Disease	No disease
Positive	true positive	false positive
Negative	false negative	true negative

$$\text{Sensitivity} = \frac{\text{Number of true positives}}{\text{Number of true positives and false negatives}} \times 100$$

$$= \% \text{ true positives}$$

Sensitivity is equivalent to detection rate.

$$\text{Specificity} = \frac{\text{Number of true negatives}}{\text{Number of true negatives and false negatives}} \times 100$$

$$= \% \text{ true negatives}$$

The following mnemonic is helpful:
Sp IN Sn OUT
Specificity = IN (positive test result in the presence of high specificity rules in the diagnosis)
Sensitivity = OUT (negative test result in the presence of high sensitivity rules out the diagnosis).

$$\text{Positive predictive value} = \frac{TP}{TP + FP} \times 100$$

Probability of disease in case with a positive test result

$$\text{Negative predictive value} = \frac{TN}{TN + FN} \times 100$$

Probability of disease in case with a negative test result
Odds ratio = Estimated relative risk

$$= \frac{\text{Odds of cases (those with disease) being exposed to risk factor}}{\text{Odds of controls being exposed to risk factor}}$$

With odds, the denominator does not include the numerator.

$$\text{Relative risk} = \frac{\text{The probability of an event in the active group}}{\text{The probability of the event in the control group}}$$

Receiver operating characteristic curve

Features

- A type of graph for assessing the ability of a quantitative diagnostic or screening test or algorithm to discriminate between affected and healthy individuals. It applies to tests with a variable cut-off point, on an ordinal or interval scale of measurement. It demonstrates the relationship between sensitivity, specificity and the choice of cut-off point.
- A ROC curve displays the relationship between the true positive rate (on the vertical or y axis) and the false positive rate (on the horizontal or x axis), i.e. sensitivity versus (1 – specificity). There is always a trade off between sensitivity and specificity of a diagnostic test.
- The true positive rate and false positive rate for each decision threshold, or cut-off point, for which data are available are plotted separately. The points are connected using regression methodology. The cut-off points may be continuous or categorical.
- The area below the curve is a measure of the validity (i.e. diagnostic or predictive efficiency) of a screening test and should always be greater than 0.5.
- The curve is a function of all possible likelihood ratios obtained from a given test.
- It helps to choose the critical value (cut-off point) at which a predictor best discriminates between choices, i.e. positive and negative. The critical value is found as the value at which the curve's deviation from the diagonal line from (0,0)(lower left) to (1,1)(upper right) is the greatest, i.e. at or near the shoulder of the curve.
- As the curve approaches the left corner of the co-ordinate system, the test performance gets better.
- The use of ROC curves helps in choosing between competing tests, especially in clinical laboratory testing and in diagnostic imaging.
- The curve takes no account of the prevalence of the disease being tested for.

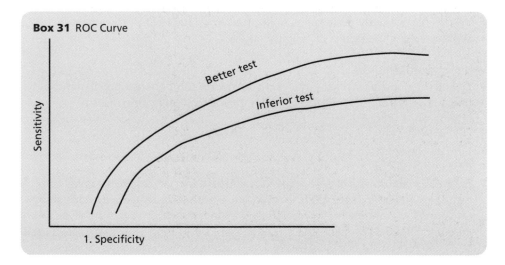

Box 31 ROC Curve

Better test

Inferior test

Sensitivity

1. Specificity

Hierarchy of clinical evidence

Ia   Strong evidence from at least one systematic review: meta-analysis of randomised controlled clinical trials.

Ib   Strong evidence from at least one randomised controlled trial.

IIa   Evidence from at least one well-designed controlled study without randomisation.

IIb   Evidence from at least one well-designed quasi-experimental study.

III   Evidence from at least one well-designed non-experimental descriptive study, e.g. comparative studies, correlation studies and case-control studies.

IV   Expert opinion: reports of expert committees, opinions of respected authorities based on clinical experience.

The Cochrane Library (www.cochrane.org) is a major source of higher level evidence via the following databases:

- The Cochrane Database of Systematic Reviews.
- The Cochrane Controlled Trials Register.
- Database of Abstracts of Reviews of Effectiveness.
- The Cochrane Methodology Register.

Meta-analysis

Meta-analysis refers to the use of formal statistical techniques to sum up the quantitative evidence from separate studies designed to investigate the same hypothesis. It improves the power of the investigations and increases the precision of the estimates of treatment effects.

It involves the combination of measures of treatment difference (e.g. differences of means, or of proportions, or log-odds ratios – which have a distribution much closer to Normal than the odds ratio itself) into a good estimator of assumed common underlying treatment effect.

Indications for considering meta-analysis
- Definitive randomised trials are impossible or impractical.
- Results of previously performed randomised trials are inconclusive or conflicting.
- While awaiting the results of definitive studies.

Steps in meta-analysis
- Define the question, which includes the following components: population; study intervention (treatment; screening; risk factor alteration); comparison intervention; outcome(s).
- Define the inclusion criteria for studies to be analysed.
- Find all eligible studies.
- Review the methods and results of each study.
- Summarise the results of each study in a standard format, displaying point estimates and confidence intervals. Calculate a **summary statistic** for each study (in general, the endpoint of clinical trials is a binary variable, e.g. dead/alive, cured/not cured). The odds ratio is used to summarise randomised controlled trials and case-control studies. Relative risks are used to summarise cohort studies.

- A **weighted average** of the summary statistics provides the overall treatment effect.
- Assess variation between studies in terms of the consistency of treatment effect (**heterogeneity**). Each of the individual study results is compared with the summary estimate. The heterogeneity statistics produce a chi-square value for each individual study, based on the comparison of that study's result to the summary result.
- Explore heterogeneity, including examination of subgroup results in the aggregate of studies.
- Interpret and report findings.

Criteria used for determining eligibility for study inclusion
- Types of study design.
- Years of publication.
- Languages.
- Restrictions due to sample size or follow-up.
- Similarity of treatments and/or exposure.
- Completeness of information.

Requirements for pooling trials
The trials should test the same hypothesis, comparing similar patients (diagnosis, age, sex, stage of disease, comorbidity) or similar interventions (drugs, doses, operations), and measuring the same outcome or endpoint (survival, wellbeing, physiological function).

Difficulties in pooling trials relate to differences among:
- Therapies: treatment and control interventions.
- Study designs.
- Patient populations: differences in inclusion and exclusion criteria.
- Follow-up times.
- Variations in analysis: handling withdrawals, drop-outs, and crossovers.
- Quality of studies.

Methods of summarising treatment effects
- Binary outcome data:
  Risk ratio
  Odds ratio.
- Ordinal data:
  Log odds ratio or log hazard ratio.
- Continuous outcome data:
  Differences in means.
- Proportions:
  Likelihood ratio
  Receiver operating characteristic curves.

Box 32 Methods of meta-analysis

Model assumption	Methods	Effect measures
Fixed effects	Mantel–Haenszel	Ratio (typically odds ratio; can be applied to rate ratio and risk ratio)
	Peto	Ratio (approximates to odds ratio)
	General variance-based	Ratio (all types) and difference
Random effects	DerSimonian–Laird	Ratio (all types) and difference

Meta-analytic models

Fixed-effects model (Mantel–Haenszel and Peto methods)
- The result from each individual trial (RCT) estimates the same effect size.
- All trials are a random sample from one large common trial.
- Each RCT provides an unbiased estimate of the treatment effect.
- The model assumes that there is no heterogeneity between individual trials.
- Differences between individual trial outcomes are due to sampling variability, measured by sampling variance. Individual studies are weighted by their precision, measured by the inverse of the variance of the parameter of test accuracy, or by the number of participating subjects.
- To recapitulate, all studies are randomly sampling subjects from the same population of patients, with the same mean but with different variances.

Random-effects model (Der Simonian–Laird method)
- The results from individual trials are a random selection from a population that follows a normal distribution.
- Differences between trials result from both random error as well as from real differences between the study populations and procedures.
- The model incorporates statistical heterogeneity (study-to-study variation) into the overall estimate of an average effect.
- The weighting factor incorporates both within-study and between-study variation.
- A greater relative weight is given to smaller trials.
- The model design leads to wider confidence intervals for the weighted average than with fixed-effects models.
- Each study outcome belongs to its own sampling distribution with different means.

Equal effects model
- The effect sizes of all trials are assumed to be equal.
- The estimates of individual effect sizes are replaced by an estimate of overall effect size.
- The model gives a narrower confidence interval or more significant overall effect sizes.

With markedly heterogeneous studies, the results of fixed and random effects meta-analyses will vary considerably.

Mantel–Haenszel estimates

- These combine information from two or several 2 × 2 contingency tables.
- A test of homogeneity is first performed to verify that the population odds ratio is constant across the groups.
- A point estimate and a confidence interval are calculated for the summary odds ratio.
- The weights usually are proportional to the degree of certainty or precision of the individual estimates (or proportional to variance of each difference between the effects of two treatments for each trial).
- Large studies are usually given more weight than smaller ones.

Peto's method

- A statistical method of combining odds ratio in a meta-analysis.
- It is based on the ratio of observed to expected frequencies, obtained with the results displayed in a 2 × 2 table.

Criticisms of meta-analysis

These relate to:

- Publication bias: meta-analysis deals primarily with published studies.
- Varying quality of the studies included.
- Pooling together of heterogeneous studies.

Funnel plots

Funnel plots can be used to examine meta-analyses for publication bias or bias due to poor methodological quality of smaller studies causing exaggeration of treatment effects.

Features

- The plot is a scatter plot of relative measures of treatment effects or outcomes (risk ratio or odds ratio) of individual studies plotted on a logarithmic scale on the horizontal axis against a measure of study size (and thereby precision) on the vertical axis. These latter may include total sample size, log of sample size, or standard error or variance of the effect estimate.
- Asymmetry in the plot, i.e. a weak or missing tail of the funnel, may be due to publication bias, location bias (negative findings receiving fewer citations or featuring more frequently in the non-English literature) bias or 'small study effects'.
- In the absence of bias, the plot will resemble a symmetrical inverted funnel, with a clustering around the 'true' treatment effect.
- It requires a large number of trials in the analysis to allow depiction of an adequate funnel.

Forest plots

Forest plots are used to display the results of the individual trials that are analysed in a meta-analysis.

Features
- Squares are centred on the point estimates of the result of each study.
- A horizontal line runs through each square to show its confidence interval, usually a 95% interval.
- The overall estimate from the meta-analysis and its confidence interval are placed at the bottom, being represented as a diamond. The pooled point estimate is denoted by the centre of the diamond. The horizontal tips of the diamond represent the confidence interval.
- Significance is achieved at the set level if the diamond is clear of the line of no effect.

L'Abbe plot
This is a plot of event rates in a treated group on the vertical axis against event rates in the control group on the horizontal axis.

Estimators of a population parameter
An estimator is a sample statistic used to estimate a population parameter. Estimation is the process of assignment of a value to a population parameter based on the value of the corresponding sample statistic.

Estimators should be unbiased (the mean of the sampling distribution of sample means equals the population mean), consistent (precision of the estimate of the population parameter increases with sample size), efficient (minimal variance with repeated sampling) and sufficient (uses all the information in the sample in estimating the required population parameter). If two estimators are unbiased, one is more efficient than the other if its variance is less than the variance of the other.

According to the **Gauss–Markov theorem**, least square estimators have the smallest standard deviation of all unbiased estimators that are linear functions of the dependent variable.

Point estimate
This is a single numerical value of a sample statistic, used to estimate the corresponding population parameter, which can be regarded as the most plausible value of the parameter. It, however, does not explicitly state the precision of the estimate. The estimate is said to be an unbiased estimator if its sampling distribution is always centred at the true value of the parameter.

p *value*
The probability of obtaining a result as extreme or more extreme than the value of the test statistic, given that the null hypothesis is not rejected, if the dissimilarity is entirely due to chance alone. It is the smallest level of significance at which the null hypothesis can be rejected. Wherever possible, the actual computed value should be reported.

The *p* value is an estimation of the degree to which the result is representative of the population.

Commonly selected *p* values are arbitrary choices based on general research experience.

A *p* level of 0.001 may represent a trivial population effect in a large sample size, a powerful population effect in a moderate sample size or a massive population effect with a small sample. Putting it in context, small differences between large groups may be statistically significant but clinically unimportant, while large differences between small groups may be clinically important but not achieve statistical significance.

Interval estimate

Two numerical values defining a range of values with a specified high probability of containing the population parameter.

The width of the interval indicates the precision, or accuracy, of the point estimate of the true value of the parameter. It acknowledges that the parameter's value is uncertain.

Confidence interval

It is an interval estimate of the population mean, which provides information about significance and the size and direction of effect of a treatment under consideration, compared with the control. It is represented by a range of values, which includes the parameter being estimated, with a specified and stated probability. It is always symmetrical about the arithmetic mean.

The interval estimates sampling variation.

Box 33 General form for interval estimate of population mean

Sample statistic (estimator) $\pm$ critical value $\times$ standard error of means

95% CI = $X \pm 1.965$ SEM
99% CI = $X \pm 2.58$ SEM
90% CI = $X \pm 1.65$ SEM

This calculation assumes that the estimate is normally distributed about the parameter value.

The confidence interval narrows as:

- Sample size increases.
- The variability of the data decreases.
- The degree of confidence required for the population mean decreases.

A wide confidence interval indicates a large degree of sampling error.

The confidence interval is measured in clinically meaningful units and provides information about both clinical and statistical significance.

The confidence level is the probability value $1-\alpha$ associated with a confidence interval.

Confidence intervals can be constructed for most common statistical estimators or comparators, including differences between means or proportions, a single proportion or percentage, relative risks, odds ratios and the number needed to treat.

Box 34 Confidence interval calculation

- Take a sample of size n randomly
- Calculate its mean x and standard deviation s.
- If an estimate of the population mean μ is to be made with 95% confidence, the upper and lower confidence limits are given by:
  $x + 1.96\ s/\sqrt{n}$
  $x - 1.96\ s/\sqrt{n}$
- The confidence interval is given by $x \pm z\ s/\sqrt{n}$, where z is the confidence level (1.96 in the case of 95% confidence)

Confidence intervals for single mean or proportion provide information about both magnitude and its variability.

Confidence intervals on a difference of means or proportions provide information about the size of an effect and its uncertainty.

A 5% significance level is associated with a 5% chance of type II error. With normal sampling distribution, this probability level comes at ± 2 standard errors from the mean.

Maximum likelihood estimation

The likelihood function is an indicator of how likely the observed function is as a function of the possible parameter values. It estimates the parameters of a population by finding the parameter values that maximise the probability of obtaining the observed sample. The best estimator is the value of the parameter under which the obtained data would have the highest probability (density) of arising.

Maximum likelihood estimators are consistent, asymptotically normal and asymptotically efficient for large samples, but often biased.

Bootstrap confidence interval for small sample size

- An iterative computer-intensive re-sampling method involving repeated simple random samples, with replacement, of the same size as the original sample from the data (sample within a sample). This allows use of a small sample, while simulating the variability that produced the data in the first place. The output of a random-number generator algorithm is used to form the bootstrap sample. The technique allows recalculation of the population parameter. In the absence of any other knowledge about a population, the distribution of values in a random sample of size n from the population is the best guide to the population. The infinite population of n observed samples, each with probability $1/n$, is used to model the unknown real population.
- The term bootstrap, arising from the concept of 'pulling oneself up by one's own bootstraps', implies a resourceful use of one's own limited resources.
- The standard error is estimated from the variability between values of the statistic derived from the different bootstrap samples.
- The assumption is made that the observed data sample is an unbiased simple random sample from the study population.
- The number of bootstrap samples required depends on the type of estimator.

- The central 95% of the bootstrap sampling distribution provides the desired confidence interval for the mean.
- The bootstrap confidence interval can be applied to any test statistic.

Monte Carlo simulation

Described by John von Neumann and Stanislaw Ulam, and named by Nicolas Metropolis, in 1949, for Monte Carlo, because of its association with roulette, a simple random number generator.

This is a numerical method for solving mathematical problems and simulating real situations that are determined by statistical processes. This is achieved by modelling random variables. It uses random numbers as a base to perform simulations of any specified situation. The uncertainty of a model's input variables can be used to generate confidence intervals for the output of the model.

One can model any process that is affected by random factors. Some a priori information about the processes to be simulated, expressed as probability distribution functions for the different processes, is required. Simulation is made by random sampling from the probability density functions. The random number generator uses algorithms from calculated seed numbers.

A **generalised Monte Carlo test** is one where:

- An observed data set is one of several possible sets.
- All possible data sets can be generated by a series of one-step changes to the data.
- The null hypothesis states that all possible data sets are equally likely to occur.
- Each possible data set is surrounded by a test statistic S.

Monte Carlo methods include:

- Importance sampling.
- Rejection sampling.
- Metropolis algorithm.
- Gibbs sampler algorithm.

Markov chain Monte Carlo methods involve a Markov process in which a sequence of states is generated, each sample having a probability distribution that depends on the previous value.

The Metropolis algorithm is a general method of Monte Carlo simulation that produces a sample by simulation of a specific Markov process with a specific equilibrium density. It allows generation of samples from the joint posterior distributions of all model parameters.

The advantages of the Monte Carlo simulation process are:

- The ability to change parameters and to investigate the effects of these changes on system performance.
- The ability to study the effects of parameters that cannot be measured experimentally.

Probability

Probability is the quantification of uncertainty, i.e. a numerical measure of the likelihood of an event occurring. It is thus used to predict outcomes. Probability can take values from 0, i.e. impossibility, to 1, i.e. certainty. The probability of an event represents the ratio of number of favourable outcomes to the total number of possible outcomes.

The complement of an event occurs when the event itself does not occur. Events are mutually exclusive when the occurrence of one event excludes the occurrence of the other. Events are independent when the occurrence of one event does not affect the probability of the other.

The sample space is defined as all possible outcomes of an experiment represented as points in the space. A sample space may be discrete or continuous.

Addition rule of probability

The probability that either mutually exclusive event A or B will occur is a sum of the probability of A and the probability of B.

Multiplication rule

When two events A and B are dependent on each other, the probability of occurrence of one event is dependent or conditional on the occurrence or non-occurrence of the other event.

The probability of simultaneous and successive occurrence of events A and B is equal to the product of the probability of event A and the probability of event A given that event B has occurred. The **conditional probability** is the probability of one event given that another related event has occurred.

A **Venn diagram** can be used to provide pictorial representation of the extent to which two or more events are mutually inclusive or exclusive. The sample space, or collection of all possible outcomes, is depicted as a rectangle. The events are drawn as circles, inside the rectangle.

Bayesian approach (inverse probability)

The Bayesian approach is a method of inference which deals with parameters as random variables having prior distributions reflecting the strength of one's beliefs about the possible values they assume, or other indirect information. The method involves adjusting the estimates of a population parameter in the light of prior probabilities. The prior probability integrated with observed data such as from a test or sample through the likelihood function yields the posterior (post-test) probability. The combined observed effect and prior probability with weighting factors are inversely proportional to the square of width of the confidence intervals. The classical or frequentist approach to statistical inference treats the parameters as fixed and non-random but unknown values. The Bayesian approach treats the parameters as unobserved random variables.

The Bayesian approach represents the first attempt to use the theory of probability as an instrument of inductive reasoning, i.e. for arguing from the sample to the population. Information arising in the course of a study is based on the observed data, and an induction of the probability of the true observation given the data available.

Bayesian methods allow for the incorporation of previously available knowledge, beliefs and information beyond that contained in the observed data to be used in the inference process. This may include data from previous studies, known characteristics of the model used, and other objective or subjective sources of data. Objections to Bayesian analysis centre around the view that the subjective selection of the posterior distribution may violate the objectivity of the data analysis.

This form of analysis is particularly helpful for identification of good diagnostic tests which permit an increase in probability of obtaining the correct diagnosis in the presence of some prior information.

The problems of this approach are:

- All possible hypotheses need to be identified and to be given a posterior probability.
- It is computationally difficult to implement.

Posterior (post-test or revised) probabilities are probabilities obtained for different possible values of the population parameter after adjusting the sample data in light of the prior probabilities.

The sum of all posterior probabilities should be 100%.

Prior (pre-test) or subjective probabilities are probabilities for the different likely values of the population parameter based on information before the new data are collected. In clinical practice this information may be derived from the history, physical signs, and additional historical and demographic data, along with subjective judgement, experience and belief. The sum of all prior probabilities should be 100%. It is inadvisable to attach probabilities of zero to uncertain events, as this will mean that there will be no influence from any data, however unlikely, to the contrary.

The usual notation for the occurrence of event A given that event B has occurred is A/B (A given B). $P(A/B)$ denotes the probability that event A will occur given that event B has occurred already. This is called the **conditional probability**.

The general form of Bayes' theorem is

$$P(A/B) = \frac{P(A) \times P(B/A)}{P(B)}$$

The **likelihood ratio** is the ratio of two likelihoods of obtaining a particular test result. It quantifies the effect of a test result on the prior probability:

Posterior odds = prior odds × likelihood ratio

Bayesian inference involves the following steps:

- Specification of a prior distribution of one or more states or parameter values.
- Determination of the likelihood of the test result obtained on the sample given some specified states or parameter values – conditional probability.
- Determination of the posterior probability.
- Decision making which is guided by the posterior probability.

Bayesian analysis is generally computationally complex, being based on a synthesis of prior, conditional and posterior probabilities.

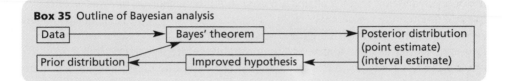

Box 35 Outline of Bayesian analysis

The most common Bayesian point estimates are the mean, median, and mode of the posterior distribution.

The Bayesian approach is useful in:

- Analysing the performance of diagnostic tests.
- Clinical decision analysis.
- The development of computer-assisted automated diagnostic algorithms.
- Analysis of forensic data.

Bayesian networks

A Bayesian network is a graphical representation of the joint probability distributions for a large set of variables. It can be constructed from either prior knowledge, observed data or both.

There are two components:

1. A directed acyclic graph in which each vertex corresponds to a random variable.
2. A collection of conditional probability distributions that describe the conditional probability of each variable.

Bayesian networks are used in expert systems, diagnostic engines and decision support systems.

Markov chains

A Markov chain is a linked sequence of random variables in which the future is conditionally independent of the past, given the present. The process can assume only a finite or countable set of states.

It represents a method of sequential analysis, where the model is used to represent time series of discrete random variables. The model predicts changes taking place over time.

A Markov chain can be considered as a random sequence of trials in which:

- Future probabilities are conditional only on the outcome in the trial immediately preceding.
- Conditional probabilities of each possible outcome are fixed.

Markov chains are used to describe stochastic processes, i.e. random processes that evolve over time. The model is useful for analysing complex problems evolving and changing over time, such as situations in which transitions can occur between a set of health states. This includes sequences characterised by recurrences of disease states and interposed treatment periods, where the transitional probability between states depends only on the current health state, irrespective of its duration and of the preceding states. Markov chains are used to study the spread of disease, and queues, among other situations.

The transitions between states are usually summarised using two matrices, the frequency state transition matrix and the probability state transition matrix. A Markov process is one in which, given a system in one state, it generates a new state of that system in random fashion.

The initial state of a Markov model is independent of the error, noise, innovation, disturbance or increments process and will have an arbitrary distribution. The transitional probability specifies the likelihoods for the system being in each of its possible states during the next time period. In a first order Markov chain the transitional probabilities of generating new states should not vary over time and should depend only on the properties of the current state and not on any other states the system has passed through. Given the present state of the system, the future is independent of the past. A Markov model has a finite memory, being forgetful of all but its most immediate past.

A two-state Markov chain is a statistical model for the persistence of binary events. A multistate Markov chain represents the time correlation of discrete variables that can take more than three values.

For higher-order Markov chains, an m-order chain is where the transition probabilities depend on the states in the previous m time periods.

Birth and death processes are Markov processes which either increase or decrease by one unit whenever there is a state change.

Decision tree

A schematic method for examining multistage decision problems which assists in identifying, organising and analysing the information that bears on a decision. Use of the method maximises the use of all component strategies. It represents a decision variable, or condition, that can vary, and determines the type of action to be taken.

Construction entails:

- Identification of the decision problem.
- Identifying all possible decisions (conditions) and events (actions) in chronological order.
- Listing all possible outcomes of the different possibilities as a series of choices, each of which is depicted by a branching point (or fork).
- Assigning probabilities to the branches arising from random nodes.
- Structuring a model of the decision.
- This comprises nodes which describe choices (patient care decisions), chances (spontaneous events), outcomes and branches.

The resultant tree structure progresses from the decision on the left to the outcomes on the right. All possible outcomes at each event are shown as branches. At each branch all probabilities range from 0 to 1.

A decision table can be used for the concise depiction of decision variables and the actions that follow. It is a two-dimensional matrix, with a horizontal row for each condition and each action, and a vertical column for each combination of conditions and resulting actions. Each vertical column is called a rule, and each rule symbolises one combination of values.

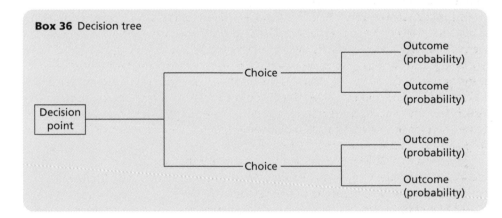

Box 36 Decision tree

Analysis of variance

This is a method of analysis for comparing the means of more than two groups, i.e. to determine whether more than two independent samples are derived from the same population. Variances are used to measure the differences among means. ANOVA is preferable to multiple *t* tests as the risk of type I error in a series of *t* tests is larger than the stated significance level (i.e. type I error probability) for each *t* test individually.

ANOVA separates the main and interaction effects of categorical independent variables (factors) on an interval-dependent variable. A main effect is the direct effect of an independent variable on the dependent variable. An interaction effect is the joint effect of two or more independent variables on the dependent variable.

There are variants for interval level control variables (analysis of covariance – ANCOVA) and for multiple dependent variables (multiple analysis of variance – MANOVA). ANCOVA allows for situations where some confounding independent variables or covariates are present, some categorical and some measured on quantitative scales.

ANOVA techniques constitute a major contribution to the field of experimental design.

The uses of ANOVA include:

- The simultaneous evaluation of the effects of multiple interrelated factors.
- Analysis of the causes of heterogeneity.

Design

ANOVA assumes that each group is an independent random sample from a normally distributed population, and that the population variances are equal.

The null hypothesis is that sample variances (and means) are equal. To test this, the *F* distribution is used. The *F* test is a test of the null hypothesis that group means on the dependent variable do not differ.

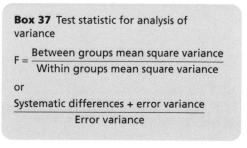

Box 37 Test statistic for analysis of variance

$$F = \frac{\text{Between groups mean square variance}}{\text{Within groups mean square variance}}$$

or

$$\frac{\text{Systematic differences + error variance}}{\text{Error variance}}$$

The F statistic takes only positive or zero values. If the computed F score is significantly greater than 1, there is more variation between groups than within groups, and the grouping variable does make a difference. If the F score is equal to or less than 1, the difference between groups is not significant and the greater is the proportion of variance due to error.

Between-groups mean square variance
- Calculate the deviation of each group mean from the total population mean.
- Square.
- Multiply by the number of scores in the group.
- Add together.
- Divide by the numbers of degrees of freedom (number of groups – 1).

Within-groups mean square variance
- Calculate the deviation of each score from its own group mean.
- Square.
- Add together.
- Divide by the number of degrees of freedom (total number of scores – number of groups).

Overall variability of responses
These can be separated into two components:

- **Variability between sample means**, indicating possible differences between population means. This may be due to either:
  Inter-individual variability
  Intra-individual variability
  Random fluctuations.
- **Variability of responses within each group**, indicating natural variability within each population: residual or error variation.

A random variable formed from the ratio of two independent chi-square variables, each divided by its degrees of freedom, is said to be an F ratio, and to follow the rule for the F distribution.

Box 38 ANOVA table

Source of variation	Degrees of freedom	Sum of squares	Mean square	F
Treatments	$k-1$	SS(Tr)	$MS(Tr) = SS(Tr)/k-1$	MS(Tr)/MSE
Experimental error	$k(n-1)$	SSE	$MSE = SSE/k(n-1)$	
Total	$kn-1$	SST		

k = Rows, n = columns, MS = mean square, MSE = mean square of errors, Tr = treatment.

One-way ANOVA

This tests differences in a single interval-dependent variable among two, three, or more groups formed by the categories of a single independent categorical variable (factor). This design thus deals with one independent variable and one dependent variable. The characteristic that differentiates between the treatments or populations from one another is the factor under study. The different treatments or populations are referred to as the levels of the factor.

Two-way ANOVA

This analyses one interval-dependent variable in terms of the categories formed by two independent categorical variables (factors), one of which may be conceived as a control variable.

Three-way ANOVA

This analyses one interval-dependent variable in terms of the categories formed by three independent categorical variables(factors).

Multivariate or *n*-way ANOVA

This test compares the population means of multiple independent variables simultaneously, while keeping the type I error at a predetermined level. The correlation among the variables is considered in the analysis. The methods available for this type of analysis include:

- Wilks' lambda: a comparison of the error variance/covariance matrix and the effect variance/covariance matrix.
- Hotelling–Lawley trace.
- Pillai–Bartlett trace.
- Roy's maximum root.

ANCOVA (analysis of covariance)

Features
- Studies the effect of one or more independent categorical variables on a single interval-dependent variable, while adjusting for the influence of other confounding categorical or interval-independent variables. These confounding variables are concomitant variables (covariates), which can be identified and measured but not controlled. This is because subjects cannot be randomly assigned to groups controlling for the covariates, as the groups already demonstrate pretreatment differences. The covariates and the dependent variable are assumed to be related. The covariates can be regarded as nuisance variables.
- The technique combines ANOVA and regression. The factor acting as the independent variable in the regression analysis is the concomitant variable or covariate. Initially, linear regression between the variate and covariate are performed. Thereafter, the *F* statistic is calculated to test the null hypothesis that all treatment effects are equal.
- Increases precision in randomised experiments.

- Adjusts for sources of bias in observational studies.
- Throws light on the nature of the treatment effect in randomised experiments.

The assumptions are:

- The covariate is not dependent on the experimental observation.
- The covariate is a fixed variable or the covariate and outcome variable have a bivariate normal distribution. The relationship between the covariate and the independent variable is the same in all study groups.
- The slopes for the regression lines within each treatment group are equal, i.e. the lines are parallel (assumption of parallelism, or of homogeneity of group differences for all values of the covariate).
- The covariate is measured without error.
- There are no unmeasured confounding variables.
- Errors inherent in each variable are independent of each other.
- The variances of errors within groups is equivalent between groups.
- The data are normally distributed.

A covariate is an independent variable that is observed and recorded, but does not determine assignment to treatment groups. It has the following properties:

- Curvilinear and linear relationship with the dependent variable.
- Curvilinear and linear relationship with the independent variable.

MANOVA model

- This involves p response variables observed for each of n subjects or experimental units.
- The response variables may be distinct variables, or be repeated measurements of either one or a set of variables.
- All response variables have the same form or are reduced to the binary form.
- Simultaneous analysis of a set of correlated response variables is possible.
- The linear relationship for each of the p response variables is described by the same set of between-unit covariates.
- The model represents an extension of the repeated measures ANOVA.

Experimental design for ANOVA techniques

- **Complete randomisation:** Completely random assignment of treatments to the subjects. This is one-way analysis of variance, there being only one source of variation involved, i.e. treatments.
- **Randomised blocks** (to control one source of error or variability): The experimental units to which treatments are assigned are subdivided into homogeneous groups (blocks), so that the number of experimental units in a block is equal to the number (or some multiple of the number) of treatments under study. Blocking controls variability between non-experimental factors in the blocks by ensuring that the experimental units in the group are similar in

some way that affects the treatment response. This is two-way analysis of variance because there are two classifications – treatments and blocks. If a block is large enough to contain replicates of treatments, the replicates are defined as block nested.

- **Latin squares** (to control two sources of error or variability): uses the Latin letters A, B, C and D.
- **Graeco-Latin squares** (to control three sources of error or variability): two Latin squares are superimposed on each other:
  The Latin letters A, B, C and D are used for one square
  The Greek letters alpha, beta, gamma and delta are used for the other square.

Latin squares design

This reduces the number of sample units (observations) required to conduct a three-factor analysis of variance. Systematic treatment bias is reduced.
The three factors in the design are:

- The factor corresponding to the horizontal rows.
- The factor corresponding to the vertical columns.
- The treatments being compared.

The arrangement of Latin letters is designed so that each letter (and thus each treatment) appears exactly once in each column and in each row.

The design permits each treatment to be applied exactly once under each level of both blocking variables, achieving a balance in the sequence of treatments applied to the blocks. Each row and each column receives each treatment once. Counterbalancing removes error variance through two-way blocking. Any variability resulting from row or column differences is eliminated from the differences between treatments. It should be used with caution if an interaction between the source of variability represented by rows and that represented by columns is suspected.

The number of degrees of freedom for the error mean square is small.

Box 39 A Latin square design for a 5×5 table:

A	B	C	D	E
B	A	E	C	D
C	D	A	E	B
D	E	B	A	C
E	C	D	B	A

Repeated measures design

The same subjects are tested with each value of the independent variable. By measuring subjects repeatedly over time, it is possible to control for biological heterogeneity between individuals.

Split-plot design

Experiments involving two factors, one of major interest B and the other of minor interest A.
Subjects are randomly assigned to the levels of factor A. A level is a treatment

category in a factor. Each subject in each level of A is tested under each of the levels of B (repeated measures design with respect to the levels of B).

Optimal experiment design
This involves consideration of the following:

- **Random allocation** of treatments to the experimental units.
- **Replication:** repetition of treatment combinations on more than one experimental unit.
- **Blocking:** allocation of experimental units to discrete groups such that the units are as equivalent as possible in relation to extraneous factors.
- **Balanced design:** every treatment combination appears an equal number of times in a block.

Diagnostic checking for a multifactorial ANOVA
- Calculate cell variances (or standard deviations).
- Assess for homogeneity of variance: Bartlett's χ^2.
- Determine the residuals from the full ANOVA.
- Check the residuals for normal distribution: skewness equal to zero; or the use of a probability plot. For smaller sample sizes (< 50), a Shapiro–Wilk test can be used to assess normality, while for larger samples the Lillefor's modification of the Kolmogorov–Smirnov test is applicable.
- Check for outliers and for patterns in the residuals.
- Look for patterns in the residuals, e.g. in time of data measurements.

If the tests indicate that the normality assumptions do not hold, transform the data and repeat the checks. If the data are not independent, transformations are generally not helpful.

Kruskal–Wallis one-way ANOVA by ranks
A non-parametric test used when different subjects are performing under three or more experimental conditions (unrelated design).

It is used to decide whether k independent samples are from different populations. It tests the null hypothesis that the k samples come from the same population or from identical populations with the same median. It requires at least ordinal measurement of the variables under study.

Method
- Rank all the observations from the three or more groups in ascending order as a single series of ranks.
- Add all the ranks together.
- Add the rank totals for each group separately to obtain a total of ranks for each experimental condition.
- Calculate the mean rank for each group.
- The H statistic gives the value of the differences between rank totals and mean ranks.

- The observed value of H should equal or be larger than the critical values from the table in order to be significant. It is an indicator of the real difference between the corresponding population medians.

Friedman two-way ANOVA by ranks

A non-parametric test used for a randomised block experimental study design where the same or matched subjects are all performing under three or more experimental conditions (related design). It is the non-parametric analogue of a two-way ANOVA.

Requirements
- The data from k matched samples are at least an ordinal scale.
- The data do not meet the parametric analysis of variance assumptions of normality and homoscedasticity.

Features
- The test is used to test the null hypothesis that the k samples (repeated measures or matched groups) have been drawn from the same population or populations with the same median.
- Since the k samples are matched, the number of cases N is the same in each of the samples.
- The same group of subjects may be studied under each of the k conditions, or N sets, each of k matched subjects are obtained, with random assignation of one subject in each set to one of the k conditions.

Procedure
- The scores for each subject for the three conditions are ranked horizontally across each row.
- The totals of ranks given to the scores within rows for each condition are added up.
- If the conditions are significantly different, the rank totals would be expected to be quite different. The column sums of ranks should be identical under the null hypothesis, indicating equal treatment effects.
- The test statistic computes the size of the difference between rank totals.
- A large value for the test statistic reflects large differences between rank totals.

Multivariate analysis

Multivariate analysis is a statistical tool for simultaneous assessment of the contribution of a number of variables, e.g. risk factors, to a single outcome.

Aims of the methods

These include:

- Reduction of dimensionality.
- Study of multivariate dependence.
- Assessment of statistical models.
- Multidimensional classification.
- Summarisation and exposure.

Classification of methods

Predict outcomes

- Multiple regression.
- Regression analysis for categorical data:
    Logistic regression
    Logit analysis
    Probit analysis.
- Canonical variate analysis.

Examining differences between groups

- Analyses of variance.
- Discriminant analysis.
- Multivariate analysis of variance (MANOVA).

Exploring underlying structure

- Factor analysis.
- Principal components analysis.
- Cluster analysis.
- Multidimensional scaling.

Discriminant analysis

- This allows objective discrimination among prespecified, well-defined groups of sampling entities based on a collection of characteristics: discriminating variables. The likelihood that an entity will belong to a group is predicted by the discriminating variables. An individual or group of individuals can be assigned to one or more known or unknown distinct populations, on the basis of observations on several characteristics of the individual or group and a sample of observations on these characteristics for the populations.
- The analysis involves situations with a single categorical dependent variable and two or more independent numerical or categorical discriminating or predictor variables.
- A variate, or **discriminant function**, is derived by linear combination of the two or more independent variables that will best discriminate between the prespecified groups. This is achieved with the smallest possible proportion of misclassifications.
- The reduction of discriminating or predictor variables can be achieved by either stepwise deletion or stepwise addition methods.
- The variate's weights are set for each variable to maximise the between-group variance relative to the within-group variance.
- The test hypothesis is that the group means of a set of independent variables for two or more groups are equal to the sum of the products obtained by multiplying each independent variable by its corresponding weight. This yields a single composite discriminant score for each individual in the analysis.
- The assumptions underlying discriminant analysis are:
  The groups of sampling entities are mutually exclusive
  Every sampling entity is measured on the same set of variables
  There are at least two sampling entities per group and at least two more sampling entities than the numbers of variables
  The independent variables follow a multivariate normal distribution
  The numbers of sampling entities in the groups need not be the same.

> **Box 40** The linear discriminant function can be represented as
>
> $$Y_{lin} = a + b1 \times 1 + b2 \times 2 + \ldots bixi$$
>
> where Y_{lin} is the discriminant score, a is a constant, $x1, x2 \ldots xi$ are predictor variables, $b1, b2, \ldots bi$ are weights (discriminant coefficients)

Analysis of multivariate structure

Methods for exploring the underlying structure of a set of variables include the analyses described below.

Factor analysis

- Detects latent structure in the relationship between variables, allowing data classification or summarisation.
- Reduces a complex set of multiple related independent variables to a smaller

data set with a fewer number of factors (or supervariables) which account for many of the original variables, being related to them in a linear manner. This represents data reduction, with loss of the original variables.

Factors are linear combinations of items, which are computed from the intervariable correlation matrix. The measure of the intervariable relationship should be product moment correlation estimates or direct estimates of covariation.

Composite variables are generated, identified and interpreted by observing their correlations or regression weights with each variable included in the analysis. These factor loadings indicate the importance of the variables to each factor.

The analysis sequentially extracts portions of variance (**eigenvalues**) to represent the proportion of variance in the data accounted for by each underlying factor. These portions get smaller as each factor is extracted. It is a variance partitioning method and requires a sample size that minimises sampling error.

A **scree plot** demonstrates the number of factors plotted against successive eigenvalues.

The number of distinct factors is assumed to be equal to the number of eigenvalues that are greater than 1.0.

Principal components analysis

- Assesses the relationship within a single set of interdependent variables.
- The principal components of the set are normalised linear combinations of the components of the set which have special properties in terms of variances.

The technique reduces p dimensions of the data set into a smaller set of new composite dimensions, where each new dimension is defined by a principal component. These new variables can be used in other multivariate techniques. 100% of the variation in the original variables is accounted for in the principal components.

Cluster analysis

Cluster analysis allows analysis of data structure – the relation of different aspects of the data to each other to allow classification.

The variables are grouped into discrete clusters (mutually exclusive groups based on the multivariate similarities among entities) with shared characteristics. Clustering methods include **partitioning or non-hierarchical methods**, in which variables are placed into relevant clusters according to the similarity they have with each other. These include optimising, density or mode-seeking, and clumping techniques. The non-hierarchical methods produce a list of clusters and their members.

The **hierarchical methods** start by placing each object into its own unique cluster and then, by examining the similarity of the objects, merging the two most similar into a new cluster. The resulting $N - 1$ clusters are examined and another merger occurs. This continues until only one cluster remains. The progress of a cluster analysis can be illustrated using a *dendrogram*, or tree diagram, where one pair of branches is joined at each step of the process as the two closest clusters are merged.

Hierarchical classification algorithms include:

- Direct optimisation algorithms.
- Agglomerative algorithms, involving stepwise amalgamation using selected clustering criteria.
- Incremental algorithms, involving successive insertion of new objects into the classification.
- Divisive algorithms, where the number of classes is increased at each step by dividing an existing class into two subclasses.

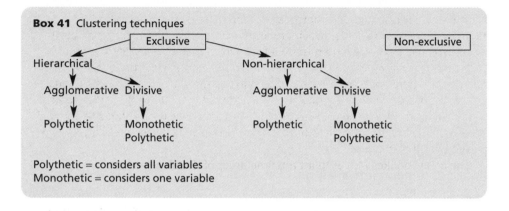

Box 41 Clustering techniques

Polythetic = considers all variables
Monothetic = considers one variable

Multidimensional scaling

Data are represented spatially by plotting variables as points in n-dimensional space. The distance between the points represents the similarity of the variables. If variable X is highly correlated with variable Y, the two variables will be situated close together on the plot.

The **Euclidean distance** between two multivariate observations is a function only of the magnitude of the distance between the points. The **Mahalanobis distance** is a measure of the distance between correlated multivariate observations. Distance measures are very useful in detecting outliers in a multivariate data set. The structure of the data can be examined in a number of ways.

Chapter 9

Time series analysis

A time series is a sequence of observations (on three or more occasions) of a random dependent variable, which are ordered in time or space. It comprises a systematic pattern and random noise (error) which may obscure the pattern.

A time series is continuous when observations are made continuously in time, and discrete when observations are only made at specific times, usually at equal intervals. Successive observations are usually dependent, allowing prediction of future values from previous observations. In deterministic time series exact prediction is possible, while in stochastic time series only partial prediction is possible from previous values.

The analysis takes into account the time order of the observations.

Uses
- Description of the properties of the series using a time plot of the observations versus time, to demonstrate the components.
- Explanation of the behaviour of the series in terms of several variables, and identification of the phenomena represented by them.
- Forecasting, or prediction of future values, of the time series variables.
- The generation of warning signals of future fluctuations, as a means of controlling the series.

Components
- Long-term or secular trend: long-term change in the mean.
- Seasonal variations: short-term and regular (periodic) fluctuations about the trend.
- Cyclical variations: long-term fluctuations about the trend, observable over an extended period of time.
- Catastrophic variations.
- Residual variations: residual, irregular or random unpredictable effects, which are not accounted for by trend, seasonal or cyclical variations.

Secular trend estimation
- Three-point method (method of semi-averages).
- The freehand method of fitting a line to the data graphically.
- Least squares method.
- Method of moving averages: This gives the same weight to all observations. The average of the most recent n observations is used as the forecast for the following period. Each new observation displaces the oldest previous observation in the set of n, resulting in the calculation of a new and thereby moving average.

- Method of weighted moving averages: Each observation receives a weight. The most recent observation usually receives the greatest weight. The weight progressively decreases for older observations.

Smoothing techniques

Methods for reducing or cancelling the random variation in a time series in order to reveal more clearly the underlying trend, seasonal and cyclical components.

- Running means: A three-point running mean replaces each observation with the mean of the observation and the two adjacent observations.
- Running medians.
- Repeated running medians.
- Exponential smoothing: Involves the automatic weighting of past data with weights that decrease exponentially with time. Greater weight is given to more recent data. The weights decline geometrically as one goes backwards in time.
- Transformation of observations.

Autoregressive models

These models can be used to summarise and model the properties of a given time series and for computation of linear predictions for estimating future values of a time series. They express the observations as a linear function of past observations in the series.

First-order autoregressive models express the current observation in a time series in terms of the previous observation and of a non-autocorrelated random variable which is unpredictable.

Second-order autoregressive models express the current observation in a time series in terms of the two most recent observations.

Autocorrelation

When observations in time series data have a natural sequential order, the correlation between successive observations is referred to as autocorrelation or serial correlation. This can be detected by plots of the residuals against time. Autocorrelation can be characterised as the serial dependence of the observations in a time series. The pattern of autocorrelation can be defined by the autocorrelation coefficients or serial correlation coefficients, which measure the correlation between observations at different times apart or time lags.

With positive autocorrelation, residuals of identical signs occur in clusters. With negative autocorrelation, residuals will alternate signs too rapidly. If no serial correlation exists, the series is said to be serially independent.

Durbin–Watson statistic

- This is used to test for positive autocorrelation in regression analysis, i.e. serial correlation among residuals.
- It is based on the assumption that successive errors in a regression model are correlated, being generated by a first-order autoregressive process observed at equally spaced time periods.

- The test statistic is based on the residuals from least squares – estimated regression.
- The values of the statistic fall in the range 0–4, with 2 indicating a random series.

Box–Jenkins models

To describe time series of continuous data a class of time series models known as Box–Jenkins models is used. The first-order autoregression model is the continuous analogue of the first-order Markov chain. In higher order autoregression models the regression equation predicting x_{t+1} can be expanded to include data values progressively further back in time as a predictor.

Delphi technique

This was developed at the Rand Corporation in the late 1940s. It is a technique for subjective or judgmental longer-term forecasting, in which a selected group of experts independently answers a sequence of questionnaires in which the responses to one questionnaire are used to produce the next questionnaire. This involves controlled feedback. The subsequent judgements of the experts are refined as more information becomes available.

The aim is to achieve consensus on an issue, with gradual formulation to a considered opinion, while avoiding direct confrontation. The description of the process should include an outline of the process whereby consensus was reached.

Chapter 10

Miscellaneous

Statistical process control

A process can be defined as a series of actions or operations that transforms inputs into outputs. Continuous quality control processes have been used extensively in the industrial setting. More recently, applications for these processes have emerged in medical practice. These include:

- Quality control for laboratory procedures.
- Performance monitoring, e.g. with operative procedures.
- Surveillance to detect any increase in rare events, e.g. congenital malformations.

The **types of procedure** available include:

- Histogram, or stem and leaf plot.
- Check sheet.
- Cause-and-effect diagram: Ishikawa's fishbone diagram.
- Pareto chart.
- Scatter diagram.
- Control chart: a graphical display of a qualitative characteristic measured or computed from a sample, plotted against the sample numbers or time. A control chart varies according to the type of data, sample size and type of control. The chart measures variability of a process over time.

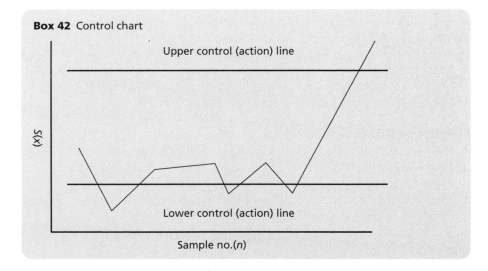

Box 42 Control chart

Upper control (action) line

Lower control (action) line

$s(x)$

Sample no.(n)

- Run chart.
- Flow diagram.

Statistical process control is primarily concerned with the use of control charts to help improve a process or a quality characteristic of a product.

The **Shewhart control chart** is a method of studying a process from a sequence of small random samples collected at regular time intervals from the process. A quality characteristic of each unit of the sample is measured and plotted against either sample number or time. The chart provides a graphical time sequence of data from the process. It comprises the following components:

- A central line representing the mean.
- Upper and lower limits or control limits, which are set at 3 standard deviations from the mean in either direction. The control limits are the limits of common cause, or the maximum expected variation of the process. Common cause variation is inherent to the process design. Data points lying outside the control limits indicate special causes. 99.73 % of the sample statistics should be within the calculated control limits when a process is in a perfect state of statistical control.
- The purpose of the chart is to determine if the process output is stable, consistent and predictable.
- The control chart will differentiate common-cause variation from special-cause variation. Special-cause variation indicates that the process is unstable, inconsistent and not predictable – this requires corrective action.

To construct the chart samples of size n are taken at regular time intervals. The statistic $S(x)$ is calculated from the sampled data. The values of $S(x)$ are plotted as they become available.

A process is in control if the control chart demonstrates the following features:

- Absence of data points lying outside the control limits.
- A similar number of data points lying above and below the central line.
- The data points fall at random above and below the central line.
- Most data points lie near the central line.

The control chart can be used in the following situations:

- To provide diagnostic information that will allow modification of the process.
- To prevent adjustment to a process that is performing adequately.
- To provide information about process capability.

Cumulative sum (cusum) method

- The cumulative sum for a series of sample observations $X1, X2, \ldots Xn$ is $Sn = \Sigma(Xo - Xi)$ where $Xi = 1$ for success and $Xi = 0$ for failure, and Xo is the reference or target value set for the level of performance.
- The cumulative sum (cusum; a measure of deviation from the target) is plotted on the y axis against the number of observations on the x axis.
- The chart is interpreted from the gradient or slope of the line joining the data points.

- A small constant deviation of the observations from the target results in the plot sloping rapidly away from the horizontal.
- A positive slope indicates that the failure rate is greater than the target value if the reference value is specified or in terms of an acceptable failure rate.
- Where the observations meet the specified criterion cusum should be relatively level, i.e. the process is in control.

The cusum method has been used for:

- The longitudinal surveillance of deaths after surgical procedures; these are plotted against the total number of operations. Application of the method requires an accepted performance standard.
- Disease surveillance procedures, e.g. to identify outbreaks of infectious diseases.

The method is more sensitive than the Shewhart chart for detecting shifts of less than about 3 standard deviations from the mean.

The **variable life-adjusted display plot** demonstrates the difference between cumulative expected mortality and actual numbers of deaths.

Models

An abstract representation of a real world physical, social or other system in terms of mathematical equations, flow diagrams, computer programs or algorithms. In statistical terms, a model describes the relationship between two or more variables. A model can be used as a predictive, a research or a theoretical tool, i.e. to predict, explore or explain respectively.

- An algorithm is a finite set of rules that provides a sequence of operations for solving a specific type of problem.
- A statistical model is a set of assumptions about the joint distribution of the data.
- The assumption is that the distribution of the data, the error distribution, comes from some specific set of distributions.
- The systematic component is a statement about the underlying pattern of the data. It is represented by a set of relations between the mean values of the data expressible in terms of a set of parameters and describing the underlying trend in the data.

Fitting is the term given to estimation of the unknown parameters of a model.

Characteristics of models
- Models are necessarily incomplete.
- The model can be changed or manipulated with ease, by changing its parameters.

Process of model building
- Formulation: simplification; representation/measurement.

> **Box 43** Scheme for a model
>
> Inputs → Process → Output

- Estimation of parameters of the model.
- Verification: checking that the model gives a good fit to the data.

Selection of the best model
The selection of the best model is guided by:

- Minimum sum of squares.
- Lack of fit tests (F tests).
- Fewest parameters (parsimony).
- Simplest functional form.
- Estimated parameter value consistent with the mechanistic premise of the model.

Types of models
- A deterministic model is one in which a given input to the model always produces the same output.
- A stochastic model is one in which a given input to the model produces an outcome which takes a range of possible values.

Validation of models
- Collection of new data, either in the same centre or preferably at another centre, to test the model.
- Split the data randomly into a derivation set and a validation set. The model is then developed on the derivation set and tested on the confirmatory set.
- Jack-knife procedure, with sequential deletion of subjects from the data set, one at a time, and recomputation of model with each subject missing once.
- Bootstrap procedure, with repeated random samples of the subjects in the data set with replacement, and averaging of the results obtained from the multiple samples.

Survival analysis – characteristics
- Studies the time taken for occurrence of a dichotomous event.
- The length of follow-up differs among participants.
- The event under study is not observed in all subjects at the end of the study. These subjects contain only partial information, and are called censored cases. The presence of censored data mandates the need for special analytical methods.

Censored observations
At the completion of a study some subjects may not have the endpoint of interest (death, relapse, etc.). This may occur with loss to follow-up, the development of an alternative outcome or voluntary withdrawal from the study. These are subjects who are removed from the database without knowledge of their survival status. Censoring assumes that if the subjects could be followed beyond the time when censored, they would have the same rate of outcome as those not censored at the time. Censored subjects are thus assumed to have the same survival characteristics of those who continue to be followed up.

Most methods assume that censoring is uninformative or only partially informative about the variable of interest.

Survival time is the time from a fixed starting point to an important event such as death, recurrence of disease or development of a symptom. With survival data analysis the special feature is the presence of subjects who have not experienced the event at the time of the study, i.e. censored subjects. Survival time can be described by three functions that are mathematically equivalent:

- The **Survivorship function** $S(t)$ characterising the proportion of individuals surviving to more than t time units, where t is measured from the start of treatment, time of diagnosis or date of randomisation, i.e. a well defined starting point. The percentage or proportion of individuals surviving to time t or beyond is expressed as a percentage or proportion.
- The **Hazard function**, or age-specific failure rate or conditional failure rate. It is the probability that an individual experiences an event in a small time interval, given survival up to the beginning of the interval. The hazard function can be estimated as the proportion of individuals experiencing the event in an interval per unit time. The function may increase, reduce, remain constant or undergo other combinations of change.
- The **Probability density function** can be used to estimate the proportion of deaths that will occur during any time interval.

The major distributions that have been proposed for modelling survival times are the exponential (and linear exponential) distribution, the Weibull distribution of extreme events and the Gompertz distribution.

There are basically two satisfactory methods for estimating $S(t)$.

Life-table or actuarial method of Berkson and Gage (1950)

- The distribution of survival times is divided into a certain number of intervals.
- The number of time intervals is selected such that the number of censored observations in any interval is small.
- For each time interval one computes the number and proportion of cases that entered the respective interval alive, the number and proportions that failed in the respective interval, and the number of cases that were lost or censored in the respective interval.
- For each interval the probability of surviving that interval is equal to 1 – probability of the event during that interval.
- The probability of an event is equal to the number of events during the interval divided by the number of cases being followed up during that interval.
- If subjects are censored during an interval, their follow-up experience is assumed to be about half of that interval. This is based on the assumption that they withdraw randomly throughout the time interval and are thus on average in the study for only half the time period of the interval.
- The overall survival probability is equal to the cumulative product of the probabilities of survival through each successive time interval. The overall risk equals 1 – the overall survival probability.

- Survival curves are depicted with an arithmetic horizontal scale and either an arithmetic or logarithmic vertical scale. The actuarial estimates are shown as a series of points connected by straight lines.

Maximum likelihood (or product limit) method of Kaplan and Meier (1958)

- This is a non-parametric technique for survival function estimation, using the exact survival time for each individual in a sample instead of grouping the times into intervals. The time intervals are between each new event and the preceding one.
- It considers survival to any point in time as a series of short vertical steps defined by the observed survival and censored times, with horizontal sections in between, providing a staircase appearance. The vertical steps indicate the times of censored observations. The steps are intervals defined by a rank ordering of the survival time. The method uses the continued product of a series of conditional probabilities, the product-limit estimates.
- Censored individuals contribute to the analysis up to the time of censoring.
- The curve is depicted by time on the horizontal or x axis and the proportion of subjects still unaffected by the hazard under study (survival rate) on the vertical or y axis.

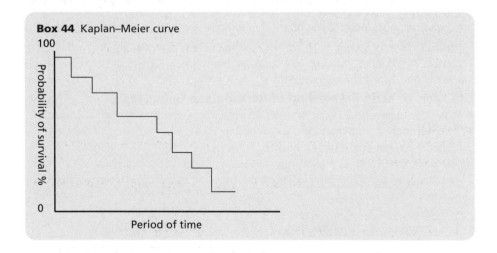

Box 44 Kaplan–Meier curve

- The product limit estimator is obtained as a product of successive survival proportions, each being the conditional probability of surviving beyond an instant of the given survival up to that time.

Survival rates can be calculated from the following data:

- All survival times in the data set, both censored and uncensored, in increasing order, from smallest to largest. An uncensored observation appears first where it has the same value as a censored observation.

- Ranks from 1 to n.
- Ranks for uncensored observations only, r.
- Computation of

$$\frac{n - r}{n - r + 1}$$

  for every ranked uncensored observation, i.e. every value of r.
- Computation of the survival rate at time t by multiplying all values obtained in the preceding step up to and including t.

A recommendation has been made recently that survival plots should include some measure of statistical uncertainty, such as standard errors or confidence intervals.

Non-parametric tests for assessing equality of survival curves

- Peto and Peto's log-rank test.
- Gehan's generalised Wilcoxon test or Breslow test: an extension of Wilcoxon's rank-sum test.
- Mantel–Haenszel chi-square test: an extension of the log-rank test.
- Cox–Mantel log-rank test.
- Cox's F test.

Regression models for estimating the relationship of multiple continuous variables to survival times

- Cox's Proportional Hazard Model.
- Cox's Proportional Hazard Model with Time-Dependent Covariates.
- Exponential Regression.
- Normal and Log-Normal Regression.
- Stratified Analyses.

Gehan test

This compares length of survival for two independent samples, and allows for censored observations.

- Every observation in one sample is compared with every sample in the second one.
- The test statistic is calculated from the difference in ranks.
- The test statistic follows an approximately normal distribution.
- The standard normal distribution is used to determine statistical significance.

Log-rank test

- This test compares two or more than two groups of survival data, or survival curves.
- The number of events in each group is compared with the expected number of events. The assumption is that all groups have the same survival rates. The test detects a difference between survival curves caused by a consistently higher event rate in one group, when the ratio of the two event rates is constant over time.

- The log-rank statistic or Mantel–Haenszel test statistic is approximately a chi-square statistic with 1 degree of freedom.

Stratified log-rank test
- This compares two or more survival curves, where the data are stratified by the effect of a qualitative confounder.
- The expected number of events is calculated separately within each stratum.

Cox's proportional hazards regression model
- A semiparametric method for assessing the association between two or more baseline independent variables and a single dependent variable, the survival time or time to the event under study.
- It assesses the simultaneous effect of several independent variables, which may be categorical (such as type of treatment received) or continuous (such as age, weight, or the dosage of drug) on survival time. The dependent variable is the logarithm of the incidence rate – the instantaneous event, or hazard, rate.
- One advantage is its applicability to quantitative prognostic factors. The technique can also adjust for confounders and for different lengths of follow-up.
- It is equivalent to multiple regression for a quantitative dependent variable or multiple logistic regression for a qualitative dependent variable.
- The model assumes that the independent variables are related to survival time by a multiplicative effect on the baseline common hazard function. There is a log–linear relationship between the independent variables and the hazard function. This means that the change in a variable results in a proportional change of the hazard on a log scale. The model provides for the assessment of covariate (independent variable) effects on the risk of an event over time. Covariates are allowed to vary over time – and adjustments can be made for time-dependent covariates, e.g. weight, blood pressure.
- Adjustments are also necessary for tied event times.
- No assumptions are made about the nature or shape of the hazard function, i.e. how the baseline disease incidence (hazard) changes over time among totally unexposed persons. It is assumed that the relative effect of any factor on the hazard function will be constant over time.
- The logarithm of the relative hazard is modelled as the sum of the individual independent variables.
- Martingale residuals are numerical values, one for each patient in a data set, that quantify the excess risk of the event not explored by the model. A large positive martingale residual corresponds to a fitted model that overestimates the risk of the event for that patient. A large negative martingale residual underestimates the risk of the event for that patient.

> **Box 45** Logarithm of Cox's proportional hazards regression model
>
> $\text{Log } \lambda(t) = Co(t) + c1x1 + \dots ck \times k$
>
> where $Co(t)$ = the hazard function up to time t; $\times 1 \dots \times k$ represent the treatment and prognostic independent variables; c is a constant.

Fradulent data

Scientific fraud is highly likely to be more widespread than reported. The reader should always be aware of its possibility, especially in evaluating study results that appear to be highly plausible in situations where there is a likelihood of uncertainty.

Types
- Data manipulation to achieve a desired result or to increase the statistical significance of findings, including selective rejection of undesired results.
- Invention of data, either fabricated or substituted for actual data.
- Plagiarism of the results of other researchers.

Features
- Larger differences between groups.
- Reduced variability of results.
- Invented extra data.

Irving Langmuir's stigmata may be used to help recognise pathological science:

- The maximum effect observed is produced by a causative agent of barely detectable intensity. The magnitude of the effect is substantially independent of the cause.
- The magnitude of the effect remains close to the limit of detectability, i.e. many measurements are necessary because of the low statistical significance of the results.
- There are claims of great accuracy.
- An epidemic of self-delusion often follows the initial description, with numerous publications on the subject ensuing.

Statistical packages

Can be menu- or icon-driven, or command-driven. They include:

- SPSS (Statistical Package for the Social Sciences) for Windows (SPSS Inc., Chicago): SPSS 11.0 (SPSS Inc., Chicago, IL 60606, USA; SPSS UK Ltd, 1st Floor, St Andrew's House, West Street, Woking, Surrey GU21 6EB, UK; www.spss.com/uk).
- MINITAB for Windows: interactive, command-driven program (Minitab Data Analysis Software, Minitab Inc., 3081 Enterprise Drive, State College, PA.16801, USA; www.minitab.com).
- Microsoft EXCEL (Microsoft Corporation, One Microsoft Way, Redmond, WA 98052, USA).
- BMDP-77 (BMDP Statistical Software Inc., 1440 Sepulveda Boulevard, Los Angeles, CA 90025, USA).
- GLIM (Generalised Linear Interactive Modelling) (Numerical Algorithms Group Ltd, Wilkinson House, Jordan Hill Road, Oxford OX2 8DR, UK).
- SAS (Statistical Analysis System)(SAS Institute Inc., SAS Campus Drive, Cary, NC 27513, USA; www.sas.com/rnd).
- SYSTAT (Systat Inc., 2902 Central Street, Evanston, ILL.60201)

www.spss.com/software/science/systat

- Stagraphics (Statistical Graphics Corpn. Inc., 2115 E Jefferson Street, Rockville, MD. 20852 USA).
- GENSTAT (Rothamsted Experimental Station, Hertfordshire)(NAG Ltd., Wilkinson House, Jordan Hill Road, Oxford OX2 8DR).
- STATA (Stata Corporation, 702 University Drive E., College Station, Texas 77840; www.stata.com).
- STATISTICA (Stat Soft, 2300 East 14th Street, Tulsa, OK 74104, USA; www.statsoftin.com).
- STATSDIRECT (StatsDirect Ltd, 11 Gresham Way, Sale, Cheshire, M33 3UY, UK; www.statsdirect.com).
- EPI-INFO 6.0 and 10.0 (Centers for Disease Control and Prevention; www.cdc.gov/epiinfo).
- PRISM 3.0 (GraphPad Software, Inc. 5755 Oberlin Drive, 110, San Diego, CA 92121, USA; www.biostatistics.com).
- GB-STAT Dynamic Microsystems, Inc. (3003 Buccaneer Road, Silver Springs, MD 20904, USA; www.gbstat.com).

The role of statistical software
- Allows data storage, display and manipulation.
- Allows file updating.
- Allows summarisation of data.
- Performs exploratory data analysis.
- Performs calculations in the application of inferential procedures.
- Connects analyses to one another.
- Allows the handling of missing data.
- Performs simulation studies.

Requirements for statistical software
- Availability of the required analyses.
- User-friendly interface.
- Flexible data entry and editing facilities. Data entry can be direct, or indirect via spreadsheets or databases.
- Good facilities for exploring data with summary statistics and graphs.
- Ability to deal with missing data.
- Ability to update and to merge data sets.
- Statistically sound procedures for fitting models and including diagnostic checking.
- Computationally efficient programmes.
- High-speed processing.
- All output clear and self explanatory.
- Easy to learn and easy to use package.
- Competitive cost.
- Adequate documentation and support from the vendor.
- Compatibility with other data analysis packages.

- Ability to customise applications.
- Ability to process large data sets where required.
- Reporting facilities.

Packages differ with respect to:

- Input requirements:
  In line
  Spreadsheet
  Separate ASCII (American Standard Code for Information Interchange) files.
- Output formats.
- Specific calculations performed.
- Algorithm used, which may lead to different results for the same test.

Among the usual features of the commonly available packages are:

- Worksheets.
- Graphics.
- Toolbars.

Problems with the use of packages relate mainly to inappropriate choice of test procedures. As the availability of statistical packages has overcome the computational problems of performing statistical tests, tests may be selected indiscriminately, thereby allowing spurious inferences from the available data.

Recommended reading/ Selected references

Recommended reading

Altman, D.G. *Practical Statistics for Medical Research*. Chapman and Hall, London, 1991.

Armitage, P. and Berry, G. *Statistical Methods in Medical Research*, 4th edition. Blackwell Scientific, Oxford, 2002.

Bland, J.M. and Peacock, J. *Statistical Questions in Evidence-based Medicine*. Oxford University Press, Oxford, 2000.

Chatfield, C. *The Analysis of Time Series. An Introduction*, 5th edition. Chapman & Hall/CRC, London, 1999.

Cox, D.R. and Oakes, D. *Analysis of Survival Data*. Chapman and Hall, London, 1984.

Everitt, B.S. and Pickles, A. *Statistical Aspects of the Design and Analysis of Clinical Trials*. Imperial College Press, London, 1999.

Freedman, D., Pisani, R. and Purves, R. *Statistics*, 3rd edition. W.W. Norton Co., New York, 1998.

Hoaglin, D.C., Mosteller, F. and Tukey, J.W. *Fundamentals of Exploratory Analysis of Variance*. Wiley, New York, 1991.

Katz, M.H. *Multivariate Analysis. A Practical Guide for Clinicians*. Cambridge University Press, Cambridge, 1999.

Kerr, A.W., Hall, H.K. and Kozub, S.A. *Doing Statistics with SPSS*. SAGE Publications, London, 2002.

Lipschutz, S. and Schiller, J. *Schaum's Outlines of Theory and Problems of Introduction to Probability and Statistics*. McGraw-Hill, London, 1998.

Long, T.A. and Secic, M. *How To Report Statistics in Medicine*. American College of Physicians, Philadelphia, 1997.

Mould, R.F. *Introductory Medical Statistics*. Institute of Physics Publishing, Bristol, 1998.

Siegel, S. and Castellan, N.J., Jr. *Non-parametric Statistics for the Behavioural Sciences*, 2nd edition. McGraw-Hill, London, 1988.

Snedecor, G.W. and Cochran, W.G. *Statistical Methods*, 3rd edition. Iowa State University Press, Ames, 1989.

Sokal, R.R. and Rohlf, F.J. *Biometry. The principles and practice of statistics in biological research*, 3rd edition. W.H. Freeman and Company, New York, 1995.

van Belle, G. *Statistical Rules of Thumb*. John Wiley & Sons, Chichester, UK, 2002.

Zaar, J.H. *Biostatistical Analysis*, 4th edition. Prentice Hall International, Upper Saddle River, NJ, 1998

Selected references

Chapter 1

Barnett, V. and Lewis, T. *Outliers in Statistical Data*, 3rd edition. John Wiley & Sons, Chichester, 1994.

Cronbach, L.J. Coefficient alpha and the internal structure of tests. *Psychometrika*, 1951;16:299–334.

Guiloff, R.J. (ed.). *Clinical Trials in Neurology*. Springer-Verlag, London, 2001.

Hoaglin, D.C., Mosteller, F. and Tukey, J.W. *Understanding Robust and Exploratory Data Analysis*. New York: Wiley, 1983.

Sturges, H.A. The choice of class interval. *J. Am. Stat. Assoc.*, 1926;21:65.

Tukey, J.W. *Exploratory Data Analysis*. Addison-Wesley, Reading, MA, 1977.

Chapter 2

Box, G.E.P. and Cox, D.R. An analysis of transformations. *J. R. Stat. Assoc., Ser. B*, 1964;26:211.

Kolmogorov, A.N. Sulla Determinazione Empirial di una Legge di Distribuizione. *Giornale dell' Institute Italiano degli Altuari*, 1933;4:83–91.

Lilliefors, H.W. On the Kolmogorov–Smirnov test for normality with mean and variance unknown. *J. Am. Stat. Assoc.*, 1967;62:399–402.

Pearson, K. Historical note on the origin of the normal curve of errors. *Biometrika*, 1924;16:402–404.

Pearson, K. On the criterion that a given system of deviations from the probable in the case of a correlated sample of variables is such that it can be reasonably supposed to have arisen from random sampling. *Edinburgh and Dublin Philosophical Magazine and Journal of Science*, 1900;50:157–175.

Plane, D.R. and Gordon, K.R. A simple proof of the non-applicability of the central limit theorem to finite populations. *Am. Statistician*, 1982; 36:175–176.

Shapiro, S.S. and Wilk, M.B. An analysis of variance test for normality (complete samples). *Biometrika*, 1965;52:591–611.

Smirnov, N.V. Estimate of deviation between empirical distribution functions in two independent Samples. *Bulletin Moscow University*, 1939;2:3–16.

Weibull, W. A statistical distribution function of wide applicability. *J. Appl. Mech.*, 1951;18:293–297.

Chapter 3

Breiman, L., Friedman, J.H., Olshen, R.A. and Stone, C.J. *Classification and Regression Trees*. Wadsworth & Brooks, Pacific Grove, CA, 1984.

Cronbach, L.J. Coefficient alpha and the internal structure of tests. *Psychometrika*, 1951;16:299–334.

D'Agostino, R.B., Lee, M.L., Belanger, A.J., Cupples, L.A., Anderson, K. and Kannel, W.B. Relation of pooled logistic regression to time dependent Cox regression analysis: the Framingham Heart Study. *Stat. Med.*, 1990;9:1501–1515.

Galton, F. Regression towards mediocrity in hereditary stature. *J. Anthropol. Inst.*, 1886;15:246–263.

Hosmer, D.W. and Lemeshow, S. *Applied Logistic Regression*. John Wiley & Sons, Chichester, UK, 2000.

Hotelling, H. Relation between two sets of variates. *Biometrika*, 1936;28:321–377.

Kendall, M.G. A new measure of rank correlation. *Biometrika*, 1938;30:81–93.

Kendall, M.G. *Rank Correlation Methods*, 3rd edition. Griffin, London, 1963.

Nelder, J.A. and Wedderburn, R.W.M. Generalised linear models. *J. R. Stat. Soc., Ser. A*, 1972;135:370–384.

Spearman, C. The proof and measurement of association between two things. *Am. J. Psychol.*, 1904;15:72–101.

Spearman, C. Demonstration of formulae for true measures of correlation. *Am. J. Psychol.*, 1907;18:161–169.

Zhang, H. and Singer, B. Recursive partitioning in the health sciences. Springer, New York, 1999.

Chapter 4

Arbuthnot, J. An argument for divine providence taken from the constant regularities observed in the births of both sexes. *Philosophical Transactions*, 1710;27:186–190.

Bland, J.M. and Altman, D.G. Comparing methods of measurement: why plotting difference against standard method is misleading. *Lancet*, 1995;346:1985–1987.

Bland, J.M. and Altman, D.G. Statistical methods for assessing agreement between two methods of clinical measurement. *Lancet*, 1986; i: 307–310.

Bonferroni, C.E. Teoria statistica delle classi e calcolo delle probabilita. *Publcazioni del R Istituto Superiore Di Scienze Economiche e Commerciali di Firenze*, 1936;8:3–62.

Cochran, W.G. Some methods for strengthening the common chi square test. *Biometrics*, 1954;10:417–451.

Cochran, W.G. The comparison of percentages in matched samples. *Biometrika*, 1950;37:256–266.

Cohen, J. A coefficient of agreement for nominal scales. *Educ. Psychol. Measure.*, 1960;20:37–46.

Conover, W.J. Some reasons for not using the Yates continuity correction on 2 × 2 contingency tables. *J.Am.Stat.Assoc.*, 1974;69:374–376.

Duncan, D.B. Multiple range and multiple F tests. *Biometrics*, 1955;11:1–42.

Dunnett, C.W. A multiple comparison procedure for comparing several treatments with a control. *J.Am.Stat.Assoc.*, 1955;50:1096–1121.

Finney, D.J. The Fisher–Yates test of significance in 2 × 2 contingency tables. *Biometrika*, 1948;35:145–156.

Fisher, R.A. On the interpretation of c^2 from contingency tables and the calculation of P. *J. R. Stat. Soc.*, 1922;85:87–94.

Fisher, R.A. The logic of inductive inference. *J. R. Stat. Soc., Ser. A*, 1935;98:39–54.

Gossett, W.S.('Student'). The probable error of a mean. *Biometrika*, 1908; 6:1–25.

Keuls, M. The use of the studentised range in connection with the analysis of variance. *Euphytica*, 1952;1:112–122.

Krauth, J. A modification of kappa for inter-observer bias. *Biometrical J.*, 1984;4:435–445.

Lachin, J.M. Introduction to sample size determination and power analysis in clinical trials. *Control. Clin. Trials*, 1981;2:93–113.

Mann, H.R. and Whitney, D.R. On a test of whether one of two random variables is stochastically larger than the other. *Ann. Math. Stat.*, 1947;18:50–60.

McNemar, Q. Note on the sampling error of the differences between correlated proportions or percentages. *Psychometrika*, 1947;12:153–157.

Moher, D., Dulberg, C.S. and Wells, G.A. Statistical power, sample size, and their reporting in randomised controlled trials. *JAMA*, 1994;272:122–124.

Neyman, J., Pearson, E.S. Contributions to the theory of testing statistical hypotheses. *Statistical Research Memoirs*, 1936;1:1–37; 1938;2:25–37.

Neyman, J. and Pearson, E. On the problem of the most efficient tests of statistical hypotheses. *Phil. Trans. R. Soc. A*, 1933;231:289–337.

Pearson, K. On the chi square test of goodness of fit. *Biometrika*, 1922;14:186–191.

Rozeboom,W. The fallacy of the null-hypothesis significance test. *Psychol. Bull.*, 1960;57:416–428.

Scheffe, H. A method for judging all contrasts in the analysis of variance. *Biometrika*, 1953;40:87–104.

Siegel, S. and Castellan, N.J., Jr. *Nonparametric Statistics for the Behavioural Sciences*, 2nd edition. McGraw-Hill, London, 1988.

Simes, R.J. An improved Bonferroni procedure for multiple tests of significance. *Biometrika*, 1986;73:751–754.

Tukey, J.W. Computing individual means in the analysis of variance. *Biometrics*, 1949;5:99–114.

Walker, H.M. Degrees of freedom. *J. Educ. Psychol.*, 1940;31:253–269.

Whitney, D.R. A bivariate extension of the U statistic. *Ann. Math. Statist.*, 1951;22:274–282.

Wilcoxon, F. Individual comparisons by ranking methods. *Biometrics Bull.*, 1945;1:80–83.

Yates, F. Contingency tables involving small numbers and the chi square tests. *J. R. Stat. Soc., Suppl. 1*, 1934;(Series B):217–235.

Chapter 5

Abrams, K.R. Monitoring randomised controlled trials. *Br. Med. J.*, 1998;316:1183–1184.

Altman, D.G. and Bland, J.M. How to randomise. *Br. Med. J.*, 1999;319:703–704.

Altman, D. Better reporting of randomised controlled trials: the CONSORT Statement. *Br. Med. J.*, 1996;313:570–571.

Altman, D.G. Confidence intervals for numbers needed to treat. *Br. Med. J.*, 1998;317:1309–1312.

Armitage, P. and Hills, M. The two-period crossover trial. *Statistician*, 1982;31:119–131.

Assmann, S.F., Pocock, S.J., Enos, L.E. and Kasten, L.E. Subgroup analysis and other (mis)uses of baseline data in clinical trials. *Lancet*, 2000;355:1064–1069.

Beecher, H.K. The powerful placebo. *JAMA*, 1955;159:1602–1606.

Begg, C.B. and Berlin, J.A. Publication bias: a problem in interpreting medical data. *J. R. Stat. Assoc.*, 1988;(Ser A)151:419–463.

Berlin, J.A., Laird, N.M., Sacks, H.S. and Chalmers, T.C. A comparison of statistical methods for combining event rates from clinical trials. *Stat.Med.*, 1989;18:141–151.

Brown, W.A. The placebo effect. *Sci. Am.*, 1998;278:90–95.

Bulpitt, C.J. Confidence intervals. *Lancet*, 1987;i:494–497.

Chatellier, G., Zapletal, E., Lemaitre, D., Menard, J. and Degoulet, P. The number needed to treat: a clinically useful nomogram in its proper context. *Br. Med. J.*, 1996;312:426–429.

Cochran, W.G. Problems arising in the analysis of a series of similar experiments. *J. R. Stat. Soc.*, 1937;4(Suppl.):102–118.

Cook, D.J., Sackett, D.L. and Spitzer, W.O. Methodologic guidelines for systematic reviews of randomised control trials in health care from the Potsdam Consultation on Meta-Analysis. *J. Clin. Epidemiol.*, 1995;48:167–171.

Cook, R.J. and Sackett, D.L. The number needed to treat: a clinically useful measure of treatment effect. *Br. Med. J.*, 1995;310:452–454.

Davies, H.T.O., Crombie, I.K. and Tavakoli, M. When can odds ratios mislead. *Br. Med. J.*, 1998;316:989–991.

DeLong, E.R., DeLong, D.M. and Clarke-Pearson, D.L. Comparing the areas under two or more correlated receiver operating characteristic curves: a non-parametric approach. *Biometrics*, 1988;44:837–845.

Doll, R., Peto, R., Wheatley, K., Gray, R. and Sutherland, I. Mortality in relation to smoking: 40 years' observations on male British doctors. *Br. Med. J.*, 1994;309:901–911.

Donner, A. and Klar, N. *Design and Analysis of Cluster Randomisation Trials in Health Research*. Arnold, London, 2000.

Easterbrook, P.J., Berlin, J.A., Gopalan, R. and Matthews, D.R. Publication bias in clinical research. *Lancet*, 1991;337:867–872.

Efron, B. Nonparametric estimates of standard error; the jackknife, the bootstrap and other methods. *Biometrika*, 1981;68:589–599.

Efron, B. Better bootstrap confidence intervals. *J. Am. Stat. Assoc.*, 1987;82:171–185.

Egger, M., Davey Smith, G., Schneider, M. and Minder, C. Bias in meta-analysis detected by a simple, graphical test. *Br. Med. J.*, 1997;315:629–634.

Egger, M., Zellweger-Zahner, T., Schneider, M., Junker, C., Lengeler,C. and Antes, G. Language bias in randomised controlled trials published in English and German. *Lancet*, 1997;350:326–329.

Emerson, J.D. Combining estimates of the odds ratio: the state of the art. *Stat. Methods Med. Res.*, 1994;3:157–178.

Fleiss, J.L. The statistical basis of meta-analysis. *Stat. Methods Med. Res.*, 1993;2:121–145.

Galbraith, R.F. A note on graphical presentation of estimated odds ratios from several clinical trials. *Stat. Med.*,1988;7:889–894.

Galbraith, R.F. Some applications of radial plots. *J. Am. Stat. Assoc.*,1994;89:1232–1242.

Gardner, M.J. and Altman, D.G. Confidence intervals rather than *p* values: estimation rather than hypothesis testing. *Br. Med. J.*, 1986;292:746–750.

Gardner, M.J., Machin, D. and Campbell, M.J. Use of check lists in assessing the statistical content of medical studies. *Br. Med. J.*, 1986;292:810–812.

Gelber, R.D. and Goldhirsch, A. The interpretation of results from sub-set analyses within overviews of randomised clinical trials. *Stat. Med.*, 1987;6:371–388.

Geller, N.L. and Pocock, S.J. Interim analyses in randomised clinical trials: ramifications and guidelines for practitioners. *Biometrics*, 1987;43:213–223.

Geman, S. and Geman, D. Stochastic relaxation, Gibbs distributions and the Bayesian restoration of images. *IEEE Trans. Pattern Analysis Machine Intelligence*, 1984;6:721–741.

Glass, G.V. Primary, secondary, and meta-analysis of research. *Educ. Res.*, 1976;5:3–8.

Hanley, J.A. and McNeil, B.J. The meaning and use of the area under a receiver operating characteristic (ROC) curve. *Radiology*, 1982;143:29–36.

Healy, M.J.R. Distinguishing between 'no evidence of effect' and 'evidence of no effect' in randomised controlled trials and other comparisons. *Arch. Dis. Child.*, 1999;80:210–213.

Heimlich, M., Abrams, K.R. and Sutton, A.J. Classical and Bayesian approaches to meta-analysis of ROC curves: a comparative review. *Med. Decis. Making*, 1999;19:252–264.

Hill, A.B. The environment and disease: association and causation. *Proc. R. Soc. Med.*, 1965;58:295–300.

Hrobjartssson, A. and Gotzsche, P.C. Is the placebo powerless? An analysis of clinical trials comparing placebo with no treatment. *New Engl. J. Med.*, 2001,344.1594–1602.

Kerry, S.M. and Bland, J.M. The intraclass correlation coefficient in cluster randomisation. *Br. Med. J.*, 1998;316:1455–1460.

L'Abbe, K.A., Detsky, A.S. and O'Rourke, K. Meta-analysis in clinical research. *Ann. Intern. Med.*, 1987;107:224–233.

Lasagna, L. The placebo effect. *J. Allergy Clin. Immunol.*, 1986;78:161–165.

Lewis, S. and Clarke, M. Forest plots: trying to see the wood and the trees. *Br. Med. J.*, 2001;322:1479–1480.

Medical Research Council. Streptomycin treatment of pulmonary tuberculosis. *Br. Med. J.*, 1948;ii:769–782.

Metropolis, N., Rosenbluth, A.W., Rosenbluth, M.N., Teller, A.H. and Teller, E. Equations of state calculations by fast computing machines. *J. Chem. Physics*, 1953;21:1087–1091.

Moses, L.E., Shapiro, D. and Littenberg, B. Combining independent studies of a diagnostic test into a summary ROC curve: data-analytic approaches and some additional considerations. *Stat. Med.*, 1993;12:293–316.

Oxman, A.D. and Guyatt, G.H. A consumers guide to subgroup analyses. *Ann. Intern. Med.*,1992;116:78–84.

Pearson, K. Report on certain enteric fever inoculation statistics. *Br. Med. J.*, 1904;3:1243–1246.

Pocock, S.J. When to stop a clinical trial. *Br. Med. J.*, 1992;305:235–240.

Sacks, H., Chalmers, T.C. and Smith, H., Jr. Randomised versus historical controls for clinical trials. *Am. J. Med.*, 1982;72:233–240.

Sacks, H.S., Berrier, J., Reitman, D., Ancona-Berk, V.A. and Chalmers, T.C. Meta-analyses of randomised controlled trials. *New Engl. J. Med.*, 1987;316:450–455.

Simon, R. Confidence intervals for reporting results of clinical trials. *Ann. Intern. Med.*, 1986;109:429–435.

Simpson, E.H. The interpretation of interaction in contingency tables. *J. R. Stat. Assoc., Series B*, 1951;2:238–241.

Smeeth, L., Haines, A. and Ebrahim, S. Numbers needed to treat derived from meta-analyses – sometimes informative, usually misleading. *Br. Med. J.*,1999; 318:1548–1551.

Smith, M.L. and Glass, G.V. Meta-analysis of psychotherapy outcome studies. *Am.Psychol.*, 1976;32:752–760.

Smith, T.C., Spiegelhalter, D.J. and Thomas, A. Bayesian approaches to random-effects meta analysis: a comparative study. *Stats. Med.*,1995;14:2685–2699.

Torgerson, D.J. Contamination in trials: is cluster randomisation the answer? *Br. Med. J.*, 2001;322:355–357.

Vandenbroucke, J.P. In defense of case reports and case series. *Ann. Intern. Med.*, 2001;134:330–334.

Yusuf, S., Wittes, J., Probstfield, J. and Tyroler, H.A. Analysis and interpretation of treatment effects in subgroups of patients in randomised clinical trials. *JAMA*, 1991;266:93–98.

Zelen, M. A new design for randomised clinical trials. *New Engl. J. Med.*, 1979;300:1242–1245.

Zelen, M. Randomised consent designs for clinical trials: an update. *Stat. Med.*, 1990;9:645–656.

Zweig, M.H. and Campbell, G. Receiver-operating characteristic (ROC) plots: a fundamental evaluation tool in clinical medicine. *Clin. Chem.*, 1993;39:561–577.

Chapter 6
Bayes, T. An essay towards solving a problem in the doctrine of chances. *Philosophical Transactions*, 1763;1iii:370–418.
Hughes, M.D. Reporting Bayesian analyses of clinical trials. *Stat.Med.*,1993;12:1651–1653.
Lewis, R.J. and Wears, R.L. An introduction to the Bayesian analysis of clinical trials. *Ann.Emerg.Med.*, 1993;22:1328–1336.
Sonnenberg, F.A. and Beck, J.R. Markov models in medical decision making: a practical guide. *Med. Decis. Making*, 1993;13:322–338.

Chapter 7
Bartlett, M. Properties of sufficiency and statistical tests. *Proc. R. Soc.*, 1937;A,160: 268–282.
Fisher, R.A. *The Design of Experiments*. Oliver & Boyd, Edinburgh, 1935.
Fisher, R.A. The use of multiple measurements in taxonomic problems. *Ann. Eugenics*, 1936;7:179–188.
Fisher, R.A. The comparison of samples with possibly unequal variances. *Ann. Eugenics*, 1939;9:174–180.
Friedman, M. The use of ranks to avoid the assumption of normality implicit in the analysis of variance. *J. Am. Stat. Assoc.*, 1937;32:675–701.
Friedman, M. A comparison of alternative tests of significance for the problem of *m* rankings. *Ann. Mathematical Stat.*, 1940;II:86–92.
Kruskal, W.H. and Wallis, W.A. Use of ranks in one-criterion variance analysis. *J. Am. Stat. Assoc.*, 1952;47:583–621.
Yates, F. and Cochran, W.G. The analysis of groups of experiments. *J. Agric. Sci.*,1938;28:556–580.

Chapter 8
Brown, G.W. Discriminant analysis. *Am. J. Dis. Child.*, 1984;138:395–399.
Kaiser, H.F. The application of electronic computers to factor analysis. *Educ. Psychol. Measurement*, 1960;20:141–151.

Chapter 9
Box, G.E.P., Jenkins, G.M. and Reincel, G.C. *Time-series Analysis, Forecasting, and Control*, 3rd edition. Prentice-Hall, Englewood Cliffs, NJ, 1994.
Chatfield, C. *The Analysis of Time Series: An Introduction*. Chapman and Hall, London, 1982.
Durbin, J. and Watson, G.S. Tests for serial correlation in least squares regression. *Biometrika*, 1950;37:409–428; 1951;38:159–178.
Jones, J. and Hunter, D. Consensus methods for medical and health services research. *Br. Med. J.*, 1995;311:376–380.

Chapter 10
Berkson, J. and Gage, R. Calculation of survival rates for cancer. *Proc. Mayo Clin.*, 1950;25:270.
Bissell, A.F. Cusum techniques for quality control. *Appl. Statist.*, 1969;18:1–30.
Bland, J.M. and Altman, D.G. Survival probabilities(the Kaplan–Meier method). *Br. Med. J.*, 1998;317:1572–1580.
Cox, D.R. Regression models and life tables. *J. R. Stat. Soc.*,1972;(Ser. B)34:187–220.
Cox, D.R. and Oakes, D. *Analysis of Survival Data*. Chapman and Hall, London,1984.
Gehan, E.A. and Thomas, D.G. The performance of some two sample tests in small samples with and without censoring. *J. Am.Stat. Assoc.*, 1969;56:127–132.
Kaplan, E.L. and Meier, P. Nonparametric estimations from incomplete observations. *J. Am. Stat. Assoc.*, 1958;53:457–481.

Kinsey, S.E., Giles, F.J. and Hulton, J. Cusum plotting of temperature charts for assessing antimicrobial treatment in neutropenic patients. *Br. Med. J.*, 1989;299:775–776.

Le, C.T. and Boen, J.R. *Health and Numbers. Basic Biostatistical Methods*. Wiley-Liss, New York, 1995, pp. 59–60.

Mohammed, M.A., Cheng, K.K., Rouse, A. and Marshall, T. Bristol, Shipman, and clinical governance: Shewhart's forgotten lessons. *Lancet*, 2001;357:463–467.

Pocock, S.J., Clayton, T.C. and Altman, D.G. Survival plot-of-times event outcomes in clinical trials: good practice and pitfalls. *Lancet*, 2002;359:1686–1689.

Shewhart, W.A. *Economic Control of Quality of Manufactured Products*. D.Van Nostrand, New York, 1931.

Steiner, S.H., Cook, R.J. and Farewell, V.T. Monitoring paired binary surgical outcomes using cumulative sum charts. *Stat. Med.*, 1999;18:69–86.

Van Rij, A.M., McDonald, R.J., Pettigrew, R.A., Putterill, M.J., Reddy, C.K. and Wright, J.J. CUSUM as an aid to early assessment of the surgical trainee. *Br. J. Surg.*, 1995;82:1500–1503.

Wells, F., Lock, S. and Farthing, M. *Fraud and Misconduct in Biomedical Research*, 3rd edition. BMJ Books, London, 2002.

Williams, S.M., Parry, B.R. and Schlup, M.T. Quality control: an application of the cusum. *Br. Med. J.*, 1992;304:1359–1361.

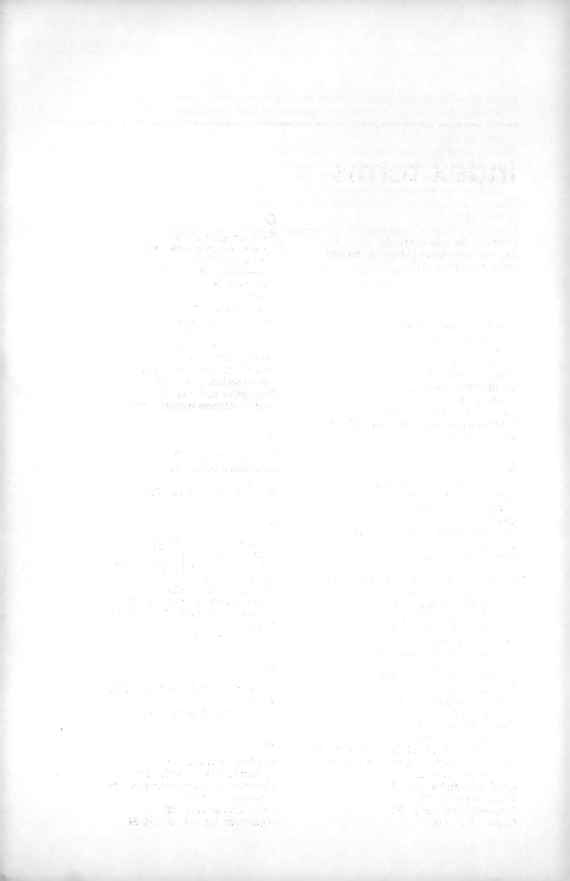

Index terms

A

Absolute risk reduction   75
Analysis of variance (ANOVA)   99–105
Autocorrelation   112

B

Bar chart   11
Bayesian theory   93–95
Berkson–Gage life table   119
Berkson's fallacy   74
Bernoulli theorem   26
Binomial distribution   25–26
Bland–Altman plot   55
Blinding   80
Bonferroni correction   58
Bootstrap confidence interval   90–91
Box and whisker plot   15

C

Canonical correlation analysis   49
Case-control study   70
  Nested case-control study   71
Causality   73
Censored observations   118–121
Census   1
Central limit theorem   31
Chebyshev's theorem   34
Chi-square distribution   33, 62, 64–68
Chi-square test   61–62
Clinical study design   69
Cluster analysis   109–110
Cluster randomisation   81
Cochran's Q   54, 63
Coefficient of variation   5–6
Cohort study   71
Confidence intervals   89–90
Confounding factors   78
Contingency tables   62
Control chart   115–116
Cook's distance   47
Correlation   37–41, 54–55
Covariates   45, 77, 99, 101–102, 121–122
Cox's proportional hazards regression
    model   121–122
Cronbach's alpha   21–22
Cross-over trial   76
Cross-sectional study   72
Cusum plot   116

D

Data, categorical   7
  collection methods   17
  nominal   7
  numerical   8
  ordinal   7
  primary   17
  secondary   17
Data transformations   34
  logarithmic   35
  modified log   35
Decision tree   96
Degrees of freedom   60–61
Delphi techniques   113
Descriptive statistics   2
Durbin–Watson statistic   112

E

Ecological study   72
Estimators, point   88
  interval   89
Experimental studies   72

F

F distribution   24, 32–33
Factor analysis   107–108
Fisher exact probability test   63
Forest plots   87–88
Fraudulent data   123
Frequency distribution   23–36
Frequency polygon   2, 10, 15, 17
Friedman test   105
Funnel plots   87

G

Generalised linear models   48–49
Graph   10, 12
Graeco-Latin squares   103

H

Hawthorne effect   79
Hazard function   119, 122
Hierarchy of clinical evidence   84
Histogram   13–17
Historical controls   80
Hypothesis testing   51, 55–56